Vagus Nerve

From Polyvagal Theory to Self-Help Practical Exercises and Diets to Unleash Your Innate Body Power and Heal Inflammation, Anxiety, Depression, PTSD, and Autism

Benjamin Corrigan

sources. Please consult a licensed professional before attempting any techniques outlined in this book.

By reading this document, the reader agrees that under no circumstances is the author responsible for any losses, direct or indirect, which are incurred as a result of the use of the information contained within this document, including, but not limited to, — errors, omissions, or inaccuracies.

Table of Contents

Introduction

Congratulations on purchasing *Vagus Nerve: From Polyvagal Theory to Self-Help Natural Exercises to Unleash Your Innate Body Power and Heal Inflammation, Anxiety, Depression, PTSD, and Autism,* and thank you for doing so. Despite the multitude of advancements in medical science that have occurred over the decades, one thing certain is that using natural methods to enhance health and prevent disease, is still the best option. Also, if we can heal ourselves with our body processes, then that's a bigger bonus. Within all of us lies the capability to improve our health outcomes and provide protection against many chronic illnesses through the strength of just one nerve. However, we won't just a nerve. The vagus nerve is a major part of the nervous system, and specifically the autonomic component. It reaches a wide array of critical areas in the body; hence, it can be used to manage the body's well-being in several ways. The vagus nerve plays a crucial role in controlling many physiological processes in a way we never imagined.

We can found several historic publications about the autonomic nervous system and vagus nerve, for example C. Darwin in 1872 acknowledged the relationship between the heart and the brain in his book *"The Expression of Emotions in Man and Animals.":*

"[...] when the heart is affected it reacts on the brain; and the state of the brain again reacts through the pneumo-gastric [vagus] nerve on the heart; so that under any excitement there will be much mutual action and reaction between these, the two most important organs of the body."

About 50 years ago, Hess in his book "Diencephalon, Autonomic and Extrapyramidal Functions" proposed that the autonomic nervous system was not solely automatic but was an integrated system with both peripheral and central neurons.

The following chapters will discuss the structure and function of the vagus nerve, as well as its place within the network. To do this, we will also detail the segments of the nervous system from top to bottom. We will get into just how large and significant the vagus nerve is and how much of an impact it has on the human body. This includes the number of physical and mental illnesses that can be prevented by maintaining its strength. It is important to keep this vital nerve functioning well and we will discuss how this is possible through natural methods and exercises that strengthen and condition the nerve. After reading this book, you will understand how to use your vagus nerve to its maximum capacity, which will allow for maximum results. There are numerous practices we will go through as there are many known methods to enhance the capabilities of the vagus nerve. Many of these techniques can be done in the comfort of your own home and will barely disrupt your activities of daily living.

It is incredible just how large of an area in the body the vagus nerve serves. The pathway it integrates through is long and crucial. Once we provide the information that we do, you will look at this nerve in a whole new light. If you did not know about this nerve before, you will now. Daily, we are affecting our health in many negative ways with practices that reduce the viability of the vagus nerve. We are here to change that and hopefully, you are too. This substantial nerve is not to be ignored and we are here to put it front and center.

There are plenty of books on this subject on the market, thanks again for choosing this one! Our goal is to provide a very comprehensive text about the vagus nerve that will answer as many questions as we possibly can. Every effort was made to ensure it is full of as much useful information as possible, please enjoy it!

Chapter 1: Knowing The Anatomy

The nervous system is a sophisticated network that consists of numerous complex structures. This network innervates every section of the body from the largest organs to the tiniest cells. The brain and spinal cord are part of the central nervous system, while the nerves, neuron, sensory organs, and any other segment that exists outside of the main framework are considered the peripheral nervous system. The two main structures of the central nervous system are where information is received, processed, evaluated, and transported. They are known as the control center that will eventually send and receive information nonstop. The information is sent through the peripheral nervous system throughout the rest of the body so that specific functions can be carried out. In simple terms, our bodies will react in certain ways to our internal and external environments. The peripheral nervous system will send the information it receives up through the nerves and back to the brain and spinal cord. These organs will then process all this information and send it back down through the nerves so the body can react as it needs to. This is a very rough overview of the nervous system. We will be describing each portion in more detail.

Consider this example: When we touch something hot with our fingertips, such as a stove, the peripheral nerves in the area sense this, and quickly shoot the information up to the central nervous system through various sensory nerve channels known as afferent fibers. Once the central nervous system receives this information, it will evaluate it and quickly send the message back through nerves through efferent fibers, telling the various structures it communicates with to move our hand immediately. This very instantaneous process highlights how quickly our nervous system functions. There is constant communication going on 24/7 that creates all of the various functions that are going on throughout the body. The circuitry and operation are quite intriguing and we will get must more detailed about all of this.

Central Nervous System

The central nervous system contains the brain and spinal cord and is the epicenter of a living organism like humans. All of the various processes occur as a result of the central nervous system and are based on what it receives and sends out. Think about it in terms of a base. At the base are the highest-ranked professionals that are receiving all of the data from outside sources. The professionals inside the base will study the data that is given to them and decide on what to do next. The professionals will then communicate this information to the people who will send it out to everyone else that will carry out the requests and demands from inside the base. The central nervous system is a highly sophisticated data processing center.

The Brain

The brain is a soft organ that is covered and protected by the skull and various forms of tissue, like the thick membrane known as the dura mater, a thinner membrane known as the pia mater and liquid known as cerebrospinal fluid. The brain is quite delicate, and if it did not have the protection that it does, it could be damaged quite easily. This organ contains about 100 billion neurons that help it operate the way it needs to. The brain is responsible for many roles of higher mental function. These include memory, consciousness, planning, and voluntary actions and movement. Besides, it controls lower body functions, like managing heart rate, blood pressure, breathing, and digestion through the various nerves that extend from it.

The brain is also quite malleable, which allows it to change continuously throughout our lifespans. When we discuss to malleability, we are referring to the various pathways that are produced by the neurons. As we gain experience and learn new things, our neural pathways will adjust and create new connections that will help us develop new thought-processes. If you look at the brain of a person 10 years apart, you will notice a significant difference. If the brain ceased to function so would all of our vital physiological processes. A few organs could function independently for a short while, but eventually, everything would shut down.

The brain can be broken down further into its various sections. Each portion of the brain tissue elicits different functions. Certain physical and mental dysfunctions can even be traced back to the area of the brain being affected based on the signs and symptoms. The brain is divided into the following sections and each one controls a different part of our living functions.

- The occipital lobe is in the posterior, or back, a portion of the brain. It is responsible for the brain's ability to recognize objects. Without this lobe, you will not know the difference between a knife and a spoon.

- The temporal lobes are located on the sides of the brain, in the area slightly higher than where our ears sit. Meaning, memory, hearing, and language are managed by this section of tissue. These lobes also interpret and process stimuli received from the auditory, or hearing, system.

- The frontal lobe is found at the front of the brain. This lobe dictates emotions, reasoning, planning, movement, and parts of speech. It is also involved in purposeful actions like problem solving, judgment, planning and creativity.

- The parietal lobes are directly behind the frontal lobe and on both sides of the brain. They are responsible for processing nerve impulses related to the various senses, like touch, taste, pain, and temperature. They even have some language functions.

- The cerebral cortex is the outermost layer of the cerebrum, which is the main portion of the brain. The cortex controls voluntary movement, reasoning, language, thinking, and perception.

- The cerebellum, below the occipital lobe, keeps us from constantly falling over. This segment controls coordination, movement, posture, and balance. Modern research also links it to thinking and emotions.

- The hypothalamus controls emotions, hunger, thirst, appetite, body temperature, digestion, and sleep. This structure is responsible for so many critical functions, even though it is the size of a pea.

- The thalamus is a motor and sensory interconnection. It receives sensory information from various sites and relays it to the cerebral cortex. The cerebral cortex also sends information to the thalamus, which relays it to the rest of the body.

- The pituitary gland controls hormones and helps turn food into energy for the body.

- The pineal gland is responsible for our individual growth and maturity. An interesting factoid is that it is controlled by light, so if a person lived in an area with literally no light, they would never grow and mature.

- The two amygdalae in your brain control your emotions like happiness and sadness. Without this structure, you would show no emotions. If you won the lottery, you wouldn't be excited, and if a loved one passed away, you wouldn't be sad.

- The hippocampus is responsible for the formation and storage of memories. Brain studies have revealed that the functioning of the hippocampus is severely reduced with Alzheimer's Disease.

- The mid-brain controls your swallowing reflexes and breathing.

- The pons is part of the hindbrain and manages motor control and sensory analysis. For example, the ears will pick up sensory information and pass it through the pons before anything else.

- The medulla oblongata lies between the pons and the spinal cord. It is the main portion of the brain stem and responsible for many body processes like breathing.

At first sight, the brain may look like a jumbled mesh of tissue, but it is a sophisticated structure that controls all of our vital functions through various networks. Our brains are evolving every day with exposure to so many new things in our environment.

The Spinal Cord

The spinal cord is a long, thin mass of bundled nervous tissue that runs down the middle of our backs. The spinal cord attaches to the posterior portion of the brain through the medulla oblongata in the brainstem. It is divided into the cervical region at the top, the thoracic region in the middle, the lumbar region below that, and then ends with the sacrum and coccyx. Just like the brain, various membranes and cerebrospinal fluid that help to protect it surround the spinal cord. In addition, hard bone structures called vertebrae create extra safety as they run down the whole spinal column. Just like the brain, the spinal cord is very fragile, so it needs a lot of protection.

The brain passes down information through the spinal cord, which ultimately gets released to the outer nerves and the spinal cord also passes information back up to the brain. The brain and the spinal cord together work to make sure the rest of the body, from our active movements, reflexes, and vital physiological processes work to keep up alive, well, and moving.

The Peripheral Nervous System

Every nerve, neuron, and sensory organ that lies outside of the central nervous system is considered part of the peripheral or outer, nervous system. Billions of pathways innervate every portion of our body and create a strong network that communicates anything and everything to and from the central nervous system. An intricate pathway that sends complicated information throughout the nervous system creates every action, movement, thought, or function. Even something as small as moving a pinky requires major communication between the muscles in this area and the central nervous system. In Summary, if the central nervous system is considered the base, every road, path, person or animal that leads back to it is the peripheral nervous system.

A Neuron

These are highly charged and excitable cells that communicate with other cells through projections known as axons. These projections communicate by transmitting electrical and chemical signals. The axons surround the cell body, which is known as the soma. The soma carries genetic information, maintains the structure of the cell, and creates energy to drive various activities. It is essentially the central nervous system of a particular cell. Neurons are often called nerve cells; however, this is a misnomer as they exist everywhere in the nervous system, and not exclusively inside of a nerve. As we mentioned before, we are born with around 100 billion neurons in our brains alone. Neurons will communicate effectively with other cells around the body through highly sophisticated channels.

Neurons are not uniform throughout the body. There are several different kinds with different actions. The following are the various neurons that exist within our nervous system.

- Sensory neurons receive stimuli from our various sensory organs, like our eyes, ears, tongue, skin, and nose. As well, they react to impulses that are generated within the body, that help to keep a physiological balance called homeostasis. An example of this is when the external temperatures get too hot and our body temperature begins rising. The sensory organs will carry a message so proper action can occur to cool down the body. This is how sweating occurs.

- Interneurons essentially act as a bridge or interlink. They receive information from the sensory neurons, process the information, and then determine if and what response is needed. They will then send this response down through the motor neurons. The interneurons are the ones in the brain and spinal cord.

- Motor neurons' jobs are to stimulate effector cells. Once these neurons receive the information from the interneurons, they will work to stimulate an effect. Once the effector cells are stimulated, they elicit the proper reaction.

We will illustrate how the various neurons work using the example of the hot stove from before. As soon as our fingertips touch the stove, the sensory neurons receive the impulse and shoot it up through the peripheral nerves. The interneurons receive the information about the hot stove, process it and determine what action needs to be taken. Once this occurs, the information is communicated to the motors neurons which stimulate the effector cells, which will cause our hand to move immediately from the heat.

There are multiple synapses or communication structures in the nervous system: that allow neurons to pass their chemical or electrical signals to their target cells. The following are examples of these synapses.

- **The neuromuscular junction:** This is a synapse between a motor neuron and a muscle fiber. Here the neuron can transmit a signal to the muscle fiber, causing it to contract.

- **The neuronal junction:** This is the site of transmission of electrical impulses between two nerve cells. This can also simply be called a synapse.

- **The neuroglandular junction:** The synapse between a neuron and a gland. Glands are organs that secrete various chemicals for use in the body or discharge into the surroundings. Adrenal glands, for example, secrete sex hormones and cortisol, which aids in the stress response.

A Nerve

A nerve is an enclosed, cable-like bundle of axons. They provide a structured pathway for the electrical and chemical impulses that travel down the axons. A single nerve consists of many layers of fibers and connective tissue that are surrounded by a single connective tissue known as the endometrium. The structure of a nerve is equivalent to an electrical cord that has multiple small wires that are surrounded by one major outer layer. The neurons would be equivalent to the electrical charges inside the cord. The nerves are essentially how information is transmitted throughout the body.

There are two categories of nerves:

- Afferent, or sensory, nerves retrieve sensory information through their receptors and send it back to the central nervous system for processing. A new sight, a familiar smell, hearing a song, touching something with your hand, or any number of sensory functions can be picked up by your afferent fibers.

- Efferent nerves are also known as motor nerves. They send signals from the central nervous system to the muscles. When you move your hand, walk, or do any other activity, those are your motors fibers at work. A common way that people remember this is that Efferent starts with an E, just like Exit. Efferent nerves exit the central nervous system.

Many of our nerves are distinctly afferent or efferent. There is also a class of nerves that contain both sensory and motor abilities. They are known as mixed nerves.

Cranial Nerves

The nerves that originate directly from the brain and brain stem are known as cranial nerves. There are a total of 12 different cranial nerves and each one comes in a pair. The different nerves carry out either sensory or motor functions, while a few of them carry out both. We will break down each of these and briefly describe their purpose.

- Cranial Nerve 1 is known as the olfactory nerve. It controls a person's sense of smell, as well as advanced aspects of taste. It is the only nerve that starts in the brain tissue. The rest originate from the brain stem.

- Cranial Nerve 2 is known as the optic nerve. Its main purpose is to transmit visual information from the retina in the eye back to the vision centers of the brain through electrical impulses.

- Cranial Nerve 3 is known as the oculomotor nerve. This nerve has both sensory and motor functions. It controls movements of the eye and upper eyelid.

- Cranial Nerve 4 is the trochlear nerve. This nerve also manages the movement of the eyes.

- Cranial Nerve 5 is known as the trigeminal nerve. This nerve actually has three different sections and each section provides a different purpose.

  - Ophthalmic Division: Provides sensation to various parts of the eye, inner nose mucosa, nose skin, the eyelid, and forehead.

  - Maxillary Division: Gives sensation to the middle third of the face, side of the nose, upper teeth, and lower eyelid.

- o Mandibular Division: Sensation to the tongue, oral mucosa, lower teeth, and lower third of the face.

  - o Side note: Trigeminal Neuralgia is a common disorder that causes severe pain and facial tics.

- Cranial Nerve 6 is known as the abducing nerve. This nerve helps to control eye abduction movement, and also gives us a sense of proprioception, which is or our body position and movement awareness.

- Cranial Nerve 7 is known as the facial nerve. It has several functions.

  - o It controls the muscles in the face that produce facial expressions.

  - o Movement of the lacrimal, submaxillary, and submandibular glands.

o   The sensation of the external ear.

o   The sensation of taste.

- Cranial Nerve 8 is known as the vestibulocochlear nerve. There are two major components of this nerve:

    o   The vestibular component helps maintain the balance of the body by allowing us to sense changes in the position of our head in relationship to gravity.

    o   The cochlear component helps us with our hearing. Cells of the inner hair and the basilar membrane determine the magnitude and frequency of sound through their vibrations.

- Cranial Nerve 9 is known as the glossopharyngeal nerve. The sensory portion retrieves information from the middle ear, throat, tonsils, and back of the tongue. The motor portion provides movement for the muscles that allow the throat to shorten and widen. This is known as the stylopharyngeus muscle.

- Cranial Nerve 10 is known as the vagus nerve. This is the longest and most dynamic of the cranial nerves and also what the backbone of what this book is about. It is fair to call it the most important single section of the peripheral nervous system. This nerve is often called the wanderer because it wanders all over the body.

- Cranial Nerve 11 is known as the accessory nerve. This nerve has both a cranial and spinal component. It controls some of the muscles in the neck and provides motor function. It also controls the muscles that allow the neck and shoulders to rotate, extend, and flex.

- Cranial Nerve 12 is known as the hypoglossal nerve. It simply provides motor function to the tongue. If the cranial nerve has a dysfunction, it can cause paralysis of the tongue.

As we can see, the different cranial nerves serve their separate functions, but also overlap with one another as well. These various nerves provide a variety of functions that serve much of the upper body. Healthcare providers can examine various cranial nerves through a battery of different tests, like pupillary reactions, peripheral vision tests, movement of the tongue, and the smell test, among others.

Spinal Nerves

31 pairs of nerves originate from the spinal cord and exit outside of holes in the vertebral column to reach their targeted tissues. These are known as spinal nerves. They control the sensory and motor functions of much of the trunk and limbs. The 31 nerves eventually branch out into countless nerve endings that innervate every portion of the periphery. Each spinal nerve has a sensory and motor root which allows for reflexive movement and conscious actions.

The spinal cord is essentially divided into five different sections: Cervical, thoracic, lumbar, sacral, and ends with the coccygeal region. Each section has its pair of nerves that serve their specific areas of the body. For example, the spinal nerves from the thoracic region cover much of the chest. While the cranial nerves innervate much of the head and vital organs of the upper body, the spinal nerves take care of the rest.

Here is a summary of the spinal nerves and the regions that they cover:

- **Cervical spinal nerves:** Eight pairs of spinal nerves originate in the cervical spine. The first three pairs help control the head and neck. Pair four control upward shoulder movement. Pair five controls the deltoids and biceps. Pair six helps control the wrist extensor muscles and also innervates part of the bicep. Pair seven controls the triceps and wrist extensor muscles. Pair eight helps control the hands.

- **Thoracic spinal nerves:** 12 pairs of nerves originate from the thoracic spinal column. The first pair controls everything on the arms from the elbow down, esophagus, and trachea. Pair two helps to control the heart, including the valves and coronary arteries. Pair three feeds the lungs, bronchial tubes, chest, and breast. Pair four feed the gallbladder and common bile duct. Pair five feeds the liver, solar plexus, and helps with general circulation. Pairs six feeds into the stomach. Pair seven feeds the pancreas and duodenum, which is the initial part of the intestines right after the stomach. Pair eight feeds into the spleen. Pair nine helps control the adrenal and suprarenal glands. Pair 10 feeds the kidneys. Pair 11 feeds the kidneys and the ureters, which are the tubes that empty the filtration from the kidneys into the bladder. Finally, Pair 12 feeds the small intestines and lymph circulation. As you can see, the thoracic spinal nerves feed a large portion of the midsection.

- **Lumbar spinal nerve:** The lumbar area covers the next five pairs of spinal nerves. Pair one covers the large intestine. Pair two covers the appendix, much of the abdomen, and upper legs. Pair three covers the sex organs, uterus, bladder, and knees. Pair four covers the prostate gland, muscles of the lower back, and the sciatic nerve. Pair five covers the lower legs, ankles, and feet.

- **Sacral spinal nerves:** The sacral spinal nerves are the next five pairs of nerves at the lower back. These pairs cover the majority of the buttocks and hip bones. The sacral nerves are the main portion of the cauda equina, which is a bundle of nerves and nerve rootlets that resemble the tail of a horse. Cauda equina is a Latin phrase and is literally translated to horsetail. The cauda equina region starts at the second lumbar nerve and finishes at the end of the spine.

- **Coccygeal spinal nerves:** The coccygeal spinal nerves are the last nerve pair at the bottom of the spinal cord and controls the rectum and anus.

As we can see, the cranial nerves control much of the cranium, and shoulder area. They overlap with the spinal nerves to cover the mid-portion. Finally, the spinal nerves cover the lower body and legs.

The cranial and spinal nerves can be assessed by testing dermatomes. A dermatome is an area of skin that is supplied by a major nerve. To test, have a person close their eyes while specific areas of the skin are tested using a pin or piece of cotton. The person doing the testing will lightly touch the dermatome, and the person being tested will tell them when and where they are being touched. They should be tested bilaterally to test both pairs of the spinal nerve. This test is often done after major spinal surgery or trauma.

With the limited number of cranial and spinal nerves, you may be wondering how these alone control every section of the body down to the most minute particle. Well, they essentially do. However, even though we only start with these main nerves, they ultimately branch out exponentially into billions of nerves that innervate every portion of our anatomy.

Peripheral Nervous System Broken Down

The outer system is broken down even further into the somatic and autonomic nervous systems. The somatic nervous system is an interconnection of nerves with the sensory receptors and voluntary skeletal muscles. Essentially, it is the section that controls the voluntary movement of the skeletal muscles. In addition, it processes sensory information that arrives from external stimuli, whether it be touch, taste, or smell.

The somatic nervous system also controls involuntary muscle movement known as the reflex arc. A reflex is a movement of a muscle resulting from a stimulus that has no input from the brain. This occurs when a nerve connects directly from a muscle to the spinal tract. Reflexes are often referred to as spinal reactions. Perhaps you have gone into the doctors and they tap you with that small rubber hammer below the kneecap, causing your leg to jerk. Maybe your muscles twitched randomly for no reason. These are all examples of the reflex arc and they are all controlled by your somatic nervous system.

Here is an example of just how complex the somatic nervous system can be. Imagine driving in your car on an open road. Suddenly, you see a large object in the middle of the road that is directly in your path. Your visual system perceives this large object and sends the information to your brain. Your brain will evaluate the information and send it back down to your muscles. At this moment, your muscles will cause you to slam on the breaks, swerve, slow down and pull over, or do whatever the appropriate action is at the moment. Thanks to your somatic nervous system, you will be able to avoid hitting that large object in the road and causing yourself major harm. The somatic nervous system plays a major part in our activities of daily living, as well as protecting us from major injuries. Without it functioning properly, we could not live the way we do.

The autonomic nervous system controls several body processes like blood pressure, heart rate, breathing, and digestion. This is the part of the nervous system that works automatically. We will delve much deeper into this system in the next chapter. Both sections of the peripheral nervous system work together to make sure all of our body processes are functioning properly. There is much more we can detail about the somatic nervous system; however, for this book, we will be focusing on our involuntary functions, and ultimately, the power of the vagus nerve.

The Connection Between The Vagus Nerve And Gut

We mentioned before about the enteric nervous system and how it's localized to the digestive tract. Well, our digestive tract has further nervous system connections due to the vagus nerve. The vagus nerve provides a direct pathway between the gut and the brain. The connection is bidirectional, meaning the communication goes both ways. For this reason, poor digestive health may have a direct impact on the central nervous system, and poor nervous system function may directly affect our digestion. In fact, many issues within the vagus nerve itself manifest themselves initially through problems in the digestive tract.

The brain-gut axis is quite intriguing. There is the adage of having a gut feeling about something. Many researchers believe that since there is a direct connection between the brain and gut, a gut feeling is quite accurate as far as sensing the environment, whether it is a person, place, the weather or anything else surrounding us. Listen to your gut the next time it is trying to tell you something.

Here is a simple linear breakdown of the nervous system.

Central Nervous System →Peripheral Nervous System →Somatic and Autonomic Components →From Autonomic →Sympathetic and Parasympathetic Components→From Parasympathetic and Partially the Sympathetic→Vagus Nerve.

Chapter 2: The Autonomic Nervous System Function

Within the autonomic nervous system lies the vagus nerve, which is the main segment. We will discuss this much further. As we mentioned previously, there are two main parts of the peripheral nervous system and the autonomic system is what controls the specific functions that we do not need to think about. These are our body processes that occur automatically based on our body's needs. If it is something we don't need to consciously control, then it is probably being controlled by our autonomic nervous system. It essentially supplies all of our internal organs and tissues. The blood vessels pushing your blood along their pathways—that is the autonomic nervous system at work. When you start salivating, that is also your autonomic nervous system at work.

Any internal physiological process that we do not need to think about is under the supervision of our autonomic nervous system. The following are the major functions that fall under this umbrella. If this system were to stop functioning, our body would fail us almost instantly.

- Digestion

- Metabolic process

- Blood pressure

- Electrolyte imbalance

- Heart rate

- Urination and defecation

- Production of many different body fluids, including saliva

- Respiratory rate and breathing in general

- Emotional responses like sadness, anger, and joy

- Body Temperature

If these processes were to cease, we would have immediate heart failure, kidney failure, as well as multiorgan failure. Our bodies would cease up and the end results would be fatal. The difference in the autonomic and somatic nervous systems can be summed up with the following scenario. When you need to run out of a burning building, your heart rate, blood pressure, and breathing rise. This is because of the autonomic nervous system. When you start running, this is controlled by your somatic nervous system.

The System Divided

The autonomic nervous system is divided further into three different sections: The sympathetic, parasympathetic, and enteric portions. All of these separate parts function in their way and their mechanisms can complement and counteract each other as needed. In the end, what makes these systems alike are the fact that they are working without our conscious mind. Many involuntary body processes are happening inside of us, that we don't realize, or even feel. We don't notice out kidneys, heart, and intestines workings, but we know that they are. The autonomic nervous system keeps us alive by controlling our most vital functions.

Sympathetic Division

The sympathetic division of the central nervous system deals with the rapid acceleration of all of the body processes. It helps to heighten our response mechanisms to unnatural levels for a limited time. It activates the fight-or-flight response. When the body perceives some type of danger, this response works as a protective mechanism to keep us out of harm's way. Multiple different hormones, like epinephrine, norepinephrine, and acetylcholine have released that help with the fight or flight response. During this period, blood pressure and heart rate rise, breathing rate increases, blood gets shunted to the peripheries, muscles tighten, pupils dilate, and digestion slows down. The body goes into full protective mode. It is ready to handle anything that comes its way, or at least put up a fighting chance.

An example of a sympathetic response is a person walking down a dark alleyway. The unknown dangers that lurk, the unusual noises being heard, and the overall unfamiliar atmosphere will create a sense of uneasiness. This will cause the various physiological responses to occur that we mentioned before. This gets the body ready for perceived danger. If something does occur, the body will be ready to react as needed. Another example is being attacked by an intruder. The body's sympathetic response kicks in and the victim of the attack is ready to fight or run away as needed. Basically, the fight or flight response is a person's safety mechanism to keep it safe in times of imminent danger.

Imagine if we did not have this response. We would have no drive or ability to save ourselves. There are countless stories out there of people performing superhuman acts when they get a major adrenaline rush and are in full fight or flight mode.

The mom who lifts a heavy object off of her child, or the hiker who fights off a dangerous animal, are all extreme examples of the strength our nervous system can give us.

While the sympathetic response is certainly heightened when fully activated, the functions of the sympathetic nervous system are always present to maintain proper blood pressure, heart rate, breathing, and other physiological responses to maintain life. Without its presence, the body would always be at a complete state of relaxation, eventually causing all of the various processes to cease function.

During this period our emotional reactivity will also become more intense. We will be prone to various emotional outbreaks and also become angrier and more aggressive. Once again, as a short-term process, this is a necessary evil. There are times in life we need to be more aggressive, assertive, and even angry. However, if we let it out of control, many different problems may occur. Negative emotions like aggression and anger can not only lead to stress and mood disorders but also lead to physical health problems down the line. Our emotions are heavily controlled by our nervous as a whole.

The sympathetic division plays a major role in reacting to any sort of stress. The early response is the aforementioned fight-or-flight. This response does not have to be related to a safety issue. Knowing that a deadline is coming up, forgetting something at home, partaking in a high-thrill activity, or working on a major project can all trigger a similar response. Everybody deals with stress on a regular basis and a short-term stress response is nothing to worry about. In certain situations, we need to have a sense of urgency and stress is critical for these moments.

The parasympathetic nervous system, which we will talk about more, is what will ultimately counteract the fight-or-flight response, and reduce stress. When stress becomes a chronic issue, that is when we have a problem. Since stress causes all of our physiological processes to go into overdrive, if we allow it to go on too long, it will eventually cause excessive wear and tear on our bodies. The continuous activation of the nervous system will eventually have negative results on a person's overall health.

People who suffer from chronic stress are at a much higher risk of heart disease, diabetes, stroke, digestive issues, mood disorders, certain cancers, and countless other long-term illnesses. People who seem to live in chronic stress are often just called drama queens. While this may be true in some instances, it could also be related to a deeper issue.

The Parasympathetic Division

The parasympathetic portion is essentially partnered up with the sympathetic division. It counteracts the responses of the sympathetic division to avoid excessive issues that can occur with a prolonged heightened response. Just like our bodies could go into a deep state of relaxation without the former and never come back, without the parasympathetic response, we would never slow down. The parasympathetic division helps conserve physical resources and maintain normal body functions. It helps to slow down the heart rate, decrease blood pressure, slow down breathing and increase our digestion, among other things. It essentially is what makes your body relax by having the opposite effect from the sympathetic nervous system on heart rate, blood pressure, and digestion. As much as we would like sometimes, our bodies cannot run on overdrive constantly. We would burn ourselves out.

After you have had a moment of extreme energy during the fight-or-flight response, you will start feeling everything slow down after a while. This is your parasympathetic response kicking in to counteract the sympathetic response. Both are crucial for helping to maintain normal body processes. Based on what it performs, the parasympathetic nervous system is often known as the rest and digest system. Our heart rate, blood pressure, and respirations decrease. Our muscles loosen up. Our mind slows down and out emotions settle. Finally, the digestive tract begins functioning normally again. Our bodies regulate our health in ways we cannot imagine.

Enteric Division

There is one more division within the autonomic system, the enteric division. This is exclusive to the digestive tract. It may be influenced by the sympathetic and parasympathetic divisions, but can also function independently of them. It is even capable of functioning independently of the brain and spinal cord. There are over 500 million neurons in the enteric nervous system and this system is embedded into the lining of the digestive tract, starting in the esophagus and extending down into the anus. Our gut essentially has a mind of its own.

Although the enteric nervous system can function alone, it mainly communicates with the central nervous system through the vagus nerve of the parasympathetic nervous system. There have been many studies that have shown the system functioning, even when the vagus nerve is severed. This system has the ability to alter its response based on many environmental factors. The following are some of the functions that the enteric nervous system controls.

- **Peristalsis:** Contraction and relaxation movements of the smooth muscle in the gastrointestinal tract. This aids in the digestion process by propelling food contents down and through the tract. Believe it or not, after we swallow our food, it does not just slide down our esophagus and into the stomach. The smooth muscles have to push it down on their own.

- **Segmentation:** This is similar to peristalsis, however, the contraction occurs in both directions, whereas with peristalsis, it occurs in just one. Segmentation allows for thorough mixing of intestinal contents, which results in greater absorption through the stomach and intestines.

- **Secretion:** This is the release of various hormones in the gastrointestinal tract that aid in digestion.

The enteric nervous system has a unique nickname: the second brain. One of the main reasons is its ability to function without the main segments of the nervous system. Besides, many of its physiological processes can mirror those of the central nervous system. Also, it consists of a diffusion barrier which is similar to the blood-brain barrier around the brain.

In summary, the autonomic nervous system functions through automatic processes through responses from the external and internal environment. We don't have to think about our nervous system functioning. It just does it on its own, based on the physiological processes it holds. There is a multitude of actions occurring inside of us regularly.

Autonomic Dysfunction

Much of this book will center around the autonomic nervous system, so it is important to understand what would happen if it did not function properly. There is a disorder known as autonomic dysfunction where the nerves of the autonomic nervous system are damaged. The problems that arise are based on how much of the system is affected and can range from mild and reversible to long-term or fatal. Some symptoms of autonomic dysfunction are:

- Dizziness and even fainting due to excessive variations in blood pressure from sitting to standing.

- An inability to alter the heart rate. Under normal circumstances, your heart rate rises significantly with exercise or other strenuous activity. If this is not occurring, there is a cause for concern. Your heart will not be able to keep up with the demands of the body.

- Sweating abnormalities, which could be sweating too much or not sweating enough.

- Bloating, diarrhea, constipation, difficulty swallowing, and many other digestive issues.

- Urinary problems like not being able to start urinating or having incontinence.

- Sexual problems in both men and women.

- Vision problems like the lack of pupillary reaction to light.

Some common diseases that can cause autonomic dysfunction are diabetes and Parkinson's disease. Uncontrolled diabetes can lead to nerve fibers losing the myelin sheaths that surround them. This significantly slows down nerve impulses. We can feel this happen with the numbness and tingling in our fingers and poor response times when it occurs in the nerves that feed our extremities. Imagine what it can do to the visceral nerves deep in our organs.

Vagus Nerve

Since we have been mentioning this frequently throughout the book, it is now time to introduce what we are really here to talk about, and that is the vagus nerve. The vagus nerve, also called the pneumogastric nerve, is officially the 10th cranial nerve. Just like the vast majority of them, it originates from the brain stem. However, while the cranial nerves innervate most of the upper body, including the shoulders, neck, and head, the vagus nerve extends well beyond the confines of this region. After leaving the brain stem, it exits through the skull through holes called foramen. It then passes through the face, neck, chest cavity, and finally ends at the gastrointestinal tract in the abdomen. It innervates all of the major organs, like the heart and lungs, as it passes through these vital areas. It also aids in many vital functions like swallowing, breathing, heart rate, and digestion.

The vagus nerve is by far the longest and most widely distributed cranial nerve. Since it also innervates several of the major organs, it is also the most crucial. This large nerve has both sensory and motor functions. The sensory functions include both somatic and superficial sensations within the skin and muscles, and visceral, which are felt in the internal organs. The sensory functions include:

- Providing somatic sensory information for the skin behind the ears, the external part of the ear canal, and certain parts of the throat.

- Providing visceral sensation to the larynx or voice box, esophagus, lungs trachea or airway, heart, and the majority of the digestive tract.

- Playing a minor role in taste sensation at the root of the tongue.

The vagus nerve also has major motor functions. This may seem confusing at first since the motor function is often synonymous with voluntary movement. However, many motor functions are automatic as well. The voluntary motor functions of the vagus nerve include:

- Stimulating the muscles of the pharynx and larynx, which deal with swallowing and voice, respectively, as well as the soft palate, which is the flesh area towards the back of the roof of the mouth.

- Stimulating the muscles of the heart. It helps to lower the resting heart rate.

- Stimulating contractions of the digestive tract, which helps to move food down the pathway.

Revisiting The Pathway

In this section, we will provide in-depth details on the pathway of the vagus nerve and explain what its main function is in each area. After learning how many sections of the body the vagus nerve effects, it will make more sense just how critical it is for our overall health and well-being. Just like every other cranial nerve, the vagus nerve comes in a pair and has a right and left section.

- The vagus nerve exits at the medulla oblongata. The auricular branch arises in the cranium, or skull, controlling the posterior ear canal and external ear.

- The nerve exits the cranium through a large hole known as a foramen, alongside cranial nerves nine and 11.

- From here, it goes into the neck and travels down alongside the carotid artery and jugular vein. At the base of the neck, the two portions of the vagus nerve go in different paths and they also split off into multiple other pathways.

    o The pharyngeal branch carries out motor control of the soft palate and pharynx.

    o The superior laryngeal branch has one section that innervates the larynx, while the other section goes to the laryngopharynx (The pharynx section that attaches to the esophagus) and part of the larynx.

- As we can see the vagus nerve plays a major part in talking and swallowing as it distributes itself throughout the neck.

- While the right and left vagus nerve disperse in different directions in the neck, they both end up in the thorax through their own pathways. The thorax is the chest cavity. Once the vagus nerve enters, the right vagus nerve forms the posterior vagal trunk, while the left vagus nerve forms the anterior vagal trunk.

- Two new branches arise in the thorax:

  o The left recurrent laryngeal nerve innervates the majority of the specific muscles of the larynx.

  o The cardiac branch regulates the heart rate and provides a visceral sensation to the organ as well.

- While the nerve does not directly innervate the lungs in the thorax, it still has a major effect on breathing and the respiratory system through its various functions. For example, the parasympathetic response helps to slow down breathing. Our respiratory tract also plays a role in vagus nerve health, which we will discuss later.

- After the thorax, the vagus nerve trunks enter the abdomen through a major opening in the diaphragm known as a hiatus. The esophagus also passes through here, and the opening can also be referred to as the esophageal hiatus.

- In the abdomen, we finally reach the endpoint as the nerve innervates the digestive organs.

Imagine the length between your brain stem and your abdomen and see for yourself just how far it stretches. Vagus is the Latin term for wandering, which is appropriate since the nerve wanders all over the body.

Ventral And Dorsal Branches

The first major division of the vagus nerve is the ventral branch and dorsal branch.

- The ventral branch is called the "feel good" branch. It sends positive messages to the brain notifying it that everything is well and good. You feel happy and active, your vital signs are at your baseline level, digestion is working properly, you are productive, and just have a positive outlook on life. When you have a positive mindset, your ventral branch is firing at all cylinders.

- The Dorsal branch is the complete opposite and causes you to be depressed. This is when your vital signs are abnormal. You will have poor digestion, feel like you're in poor overall health, and will deal with various mood disorders.

While we would like to have our ventral branch work all of the time, there will be times when your dorsal branch will be the dominant component for the day. For some people, it will be much more common. The goal is to get your ventral branch firing more often, so your mood and physical health stay good.

Later in this book, we will go over how to specifically stimulate the ventral branch of the vagus nerve.

Vasovagal Syncope

The vagus nerve has a major effect on slowing down your heart rate lowering blood pressure. In most cases, this is a protective mechanism to maintain balance. However, when the heart rate and blood pressure drop too low, it can cause a person to faint. This is known as vasovagal syncope.

Some of the common causes that trigger vasovagal syncope are:

- Standing for extended periods

- Standing up or turning around too quickly

- The site of blood and having your blood drawn

- Heat exposure

- Straining, such as with a bowel movement

With the vasovagal response, you may not always pass out but just get dizzy. If you notice this occurring, especially if you are aware of your triggers, do your best to avoid harming yourself. Lie down if you can. If not try sitting with your head between your knees. These maneuvers can help keep your heart rate and blood pressure from dropping too low.

A few signs and symptoms to look out for to prevent injury are:

- Lightheadedness

- Pale skin

- Nausea

- Feeling warm

- Excessing yawning-a big sign of low blood pressure

- Blurred vision

If you experience any of these or other signs and symptoms of an impending syncopal episode, then take the proper precautions immediately to avoid fainting completely. The vasovagal response can become a more common occurrence after someone has gone through open-heart surgery.

Disorders Of The Vagus Nerve

Since the vagus nerve is so widely distributed through many considerable areas of the body, disorders of the nerve can have serious consequences. The various signs and symptoms can also be wide-ranging Disorders of the vagus nerve are usually related to prolonged diabetes, which can slow reactionary time in the nerve, trauma or surgery, and in some cases, lesions.

Some potential clues to look out for that indicate nerve damage are:

- Impairment of speech and poor voice quality

- Inability to drink fluids

- Absent gag reflex

- Nausea and/or vomiting

- Bloating or abdominal pain

- Ear

- Heart rate abnormality

- Unusually high or low blood pressure

None of these signs or symptoms are conclusive. Much more follow up would be needed. However, they can be quite indicative of a vagus nerve disorder. Whatever the case, it is recommended that an assessment and diagnostic examinations are being done.

Gastroparesis

Gastroparesis is a condition that affects the involuntary contractions of the digestive system. Stomach contents can no longer empty properly, or even at all. Experts believe that damage to the vagus nerve can cause this to occur. Symptoms of gastroparesis include:

- Nausea and vomiting. People will often vomit hours after eating because their food will not digest properly.

- Loss of appetite or feeling full after only a few bites. Since stomach contents are not emptying, you will become full much faster.

- Acid reflux, where stomach acids are backflowing up into the esophagus. This can result in painful heartburn.

- Major fluctuations in blood sugar are common too.

Hiatal Hernia And The Vagus Nerve

A hiatal hernia is a condition in which part of your stomach bulges through the opening in your diaphragm. Your diaphragm is a muscle that separates your chest cavity from your abdomen. There is a hole just big enough for your esophagus to pass through. In some cases, the top part of your stomach will pass through this hole as well, causing the hernia. A small hernia may not create many issues; however, a large one can create many health consequences. If part of your stomach is blocked due to the hernia, it will have a major effect on digestion.

Some symptoms of a hiatal hernia include:

- Heartburn

- Nausea and vomiting

- Difficulty swallowing

- Shortness of breath (The diaphragm plays a major role in respirations)

- Chest or abdominal pain

- Acid reflux

A hiatal hernia can negatively affect the vagus nerve also. The vagus nerve passes through the same hole as the esophagus through the diaphragm to get to the abdominal cavity. When there is a hernia, it will compress the vagus nerve and cause major dysfunction. When this occurs, we will have the same health issues that result from a dysfunctional vagus nerve. In turn, further digestive, heart, breathing, and swallowing issues can manifest themselves. If you notice the signs and symptoms of a hiatal hernia, get checked out immediately.

Vagotomy

A vagotomy is a surgery that removes part or all of the vagus nerve. Vagotomy procedures used to be quite common for treating major stomach ulcers; however, with the advancement of medical science, they are not nearly as necessary any longer. Vagotomies would work because removing the vagus nerve reduced the number of stomach acids being produced. If these procedures are done now, it is usually alongside another major procedure and rarely done solo.

The Polyvagal Theory

The polyvagal theory was created and introduced by Dr. Stephen Porges in 1994. The theory intertwines the evolution of the autonomic nervous system to social behavior. In his theory, Dr. Porges emphasizes the importance of a person's physiological state in the expression of behavioral problems and disorders. We discussed earlier the relationship between the sympathetic and parasympathetic nervous systems. While the two components certainly counteract each other, Dr. Porges suggests in his theory that there is a hierarchy of responses within the autonomic nervous system, rather than an equal balance.

The hierarchy of responses relates to the evolution of the stages of the autonomic nervous system. These stages developed over time with immobilization being the most primitive. Eventually, we would develop the mobilization response, and then eventually social engagement. Here are the three stages described by Dr. Porges

- **Immobilization:** This is the oldest pathway that involves an immobilization response. The dorsal, or back portion of the vagus nerve responds to cues of extreme danger by making us freeze up and become numb. We respond to fear not by slowing down but actually stopping in our tracks. It appears as if our parasympathetic nervous system is kicking into overdrive. Think about the times you were so frightened that you literally froze and could not move. You were experiencing an immobilization response at this time.

- **Mobilization:** Dr. Porges suggests that this was the next pathway to develop in the hierarchy. During this state, we jump into action with our adrenaline rush and do what we need to escape whatever danger we are in. This can mean fighting or running for our lives. This is the fight or flight response that we spoke of earlier.

- **Social Engagement:** This is considered the newest development in our response system. The social engagement system consists of a somatomotor component (solid blocks) and a visceromotor component (dashed blocks). The somatomotor component involves special visceral efferent pathways that regulate the muscles of the face and head, while the visceromotor component involves the regulation of the heart and bronchi. This comes from our ventral, or front, side of our vagus nerve and allows us to feel anchored and safe in our current situation. This response came about as humans and mammals developed the ability to pick up on safety cues and then have the ability to express them. During the social engagement response, we will feel more engaged with our environment, including the people around us.

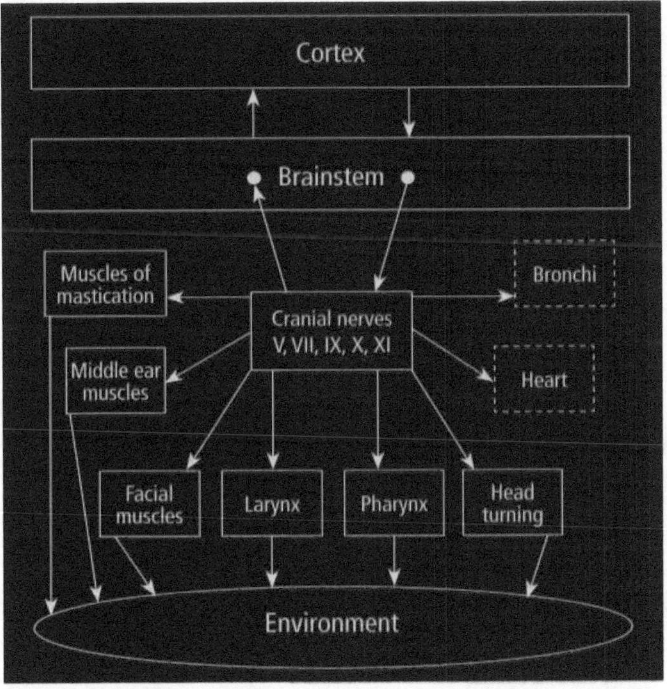

This is currently the final and most advanced stage in our evolution, according to the polyvagal theory.

The polyvagal theory suggests that we can move in and out of these phases fluidly throughout the day. As we continuously engage with our environment, there will be times where we feel safe, and times where we feel unsafe. We will have feelings of social engagement when we are near a friend or loved one, and then be in a mobilization response when we meet a hostile person. Finally, there are times that we are overwhelmed with our fears that we eventually shut down. We will be in the phase of complete mobilization at this time. For example, we may be getting attacked, but have no way of escaping, whether by fighting or running. We will simply curl up and get into a defensive position, hoping not to incur too much damage. We will make the polyvagal theory more understandable by incorporating it into real-life settings.

Trauma's Effect On The Polyvagal Theory

Any kind of trauma, whether it is physical, emotional, or mental, can have a significant effect on a person's mindset and disrupt the process of the polyvagal theory. People who have had past trauma can often be in a state of perpetual fight or flight. Furthermore, many individuals who survived trauma cannot incite a fight or flight response. These survivors will live in a state of constant shut down or immobilization. You have probably witnessed this in your own life, even within yourself. When a person is in a state of perpetual shutdown, they lose their ability to be happy, trusting, or engaged. They are essentially stuck in a primitive evolutionary state.

In counseling settings, therapists recognize these traits to help someone come out of their distress. When a person is in a constant fight or flight mindset, their bodies are always on heightened alert. This does not necessarily mean that they are moving 100 miles a minute all of the time, but they are always feeling a sense of urgency and distrust. They never have the full ability to relax. If they are sitting on the couch, they are worried about someone coming through the wall to attack them, or the roof collapsing on them. Therapists have learned to help people harness this mindset into productive activities. For example, they will clean the house, rake the leaves, or paint a portrait. Creating a sense of productivity will help people from being overcome by anxiety.

For those who are in a constant state of a shutdown have no ability in their present state to be socially engaged. They are depressed, withdrawn, and don't want to be around anybody. While this may be beneficial for them for a short-term period, long term effects of isolation are quite detrimental. Therapists and counselors have learned that they need to move people from the shutdown state into a temporary fight or flight response through various advanced techniques. Once a person is in a fight or flight response, it wakes them up, which allows further interventions to be performed. The work can start being done to move them into feeling a sense of safety. Once they feel a sense of safety, then they can be moved into social engagement.

Therapists use many body-awareness techniques to help people get out of dissociative phases. When they are in these shutdown mindsets, they will not be productive at all and will not be actively engaged in improving themselves. Once they are moved into a state of anxiety, they are more present in their bodies. After this, further thought restructuring techniques could be performed to help people evaluate their safety. Dr. Porges' polyvagal theory has been incorporated into the world of healthcare in major ways.

Healthcare workers of all types need to be cognizant of people's mindsets to take great care of them. If a person is in a state of shutdown, clinicians must recognize this to assess how to move further. When a person is in a shutdown phase, they will not be receptive to education or be interested in improving their outcomes in any way. They may go along to get along, but as far as doing any of the work themselves, this will be out of the question. Therefore, healthcare providers must also learn to recognize what mindset the patients they are caring for are in. Are they withdrawn and inattentive? Are they extremely anxious and irritable? Or, are they fully engaged and ready to take care of themselves?

Let's look at some different examples:

- Patient A is feeling depressed and just wants to be left alone. When it is time to take medications, he takes them because he is told to do so. He has no actual interest in what they are. When clinicians try to educate him, he simply does not listen and is completely withdrawn. This particular patient is not able to take care of himself at this moment. He will not be receptive to any education and certainly will not take the initiative to look after his health. Healthcare workers must recognize this as a potential problem for when the patient goes home. He will likely end up back in the hospital quickly, or worse. Interventions must be done to help move Patient A into a different mindset.

- Patient B is attentive to his health. He appears to listen when spoken to and asks many questions. However, he is quite anxious and nervous. He is certainly mindful of where he is, but unaware of all that is happening to him. Patient B must also be handled carefully. With his current mindset, he may listen, but will not be fully attentive like he needs to be. He needs to be helped to have a sense of security and safety, so he can better understand what is going on and take care of himself. Patient B is several steps ahead of Patient A, but more work needs to be done.

- Patients C is calm, relaxed, and feels completely at peace. He listens to people when they speak to him and even asks proper follow-up questions. She is active in her health and takes initiative. Patient C is in the social engagement stage and is fully aware of what is happening to him. Healthcare providers need to worry much less about Patient C than they did about Patient A and B.

Whether dealing with mental or physical health, having a positive understanding of the polyvagal theory hierarchy can be beneficial in treating patients. Being able to assess the shifts between the shutdown phase, fight or flight phase, and social engagement phase will help clinicians understand what level of functionality people are at. Having an understanding of our hierarchy can also help us determine where we are in our mindset. Knowing this will help us determine how ready we are to help ourselves.

Ventral Vagus Nerve In Relation To Polyvagal Theory

Dr. Stephen Porges chose the name Social Engagement System because the middle ear is affected by the ventral vagus nerve. The middle ear blocks excess background noise, which helps to hear human voices better. It also affects the muscles which allow facial expressions and control the larynx, which allows for proper voice quality. Simply put, the ventral vagus nerve has a major impact on our communicative processes, and in turn, our social engagement. Many people with poor social engagement have issues with their inner ears, which does not allow them to pick up on soothing sounds. Dr. Porges studied ways to improve the functioning of the middle ear through the vagus nerve to help improve the social engagement system.

Based on his knowledge of the vagus nerve, Dr. Porges also worked on ways to improve conscious breathing as a way to impact the vagus nerve positively. He found that exhaling for a longer time than inhaling helps to activate the parasympathetic nervous system, which can help bring a person from the fight or flight response to the social engagement response. These conscious deep breaths can also move a person from the shutdown response to the fight or flight response.

Social Engagement<->Fight or Flight

Fight or Flight<->Shutdown

Social Engagement<- / ->Shutdown

This simple flow chart shows that there is a direct link between the shutdown phase and the fight or flight phase; however, no direct link between shutdown and fight or flight. As living beings, we must move from top to bottom through the whole hierarchy.

Neuroception

Neuroception is a way for us to subconsciously detect threats to our safety. When we become scared, it is intuitive. We do not have to think about it; it just happens. Neuroception is another term that was coined by Dr. Stephen Porges. It is a playoff the word perception. Dr. Porges states that this ability exists in the most primitive areas of our brain, without any conscious awareness from us. All of this occurs on a much deeper level than we understand. We have our internal detection abilities to understand if a person or environment is safe or dangerous. This will trigger neurobiologically determined prosocial or defensive behaviors.

According to Dr. Porges, while we may not be aware of the presence of danger on a conscious level, we can be on a neurophysiological level. This means that our body has already started the neural processes that can lead to the eventual fight/flight/freeze responses we described above. Our nervous system is so sophisticated that it can sense danger before we even know its there. For example, we may not realize there is a threat behind us because we do not see it, hear it or sense it in any way. However, our internal neural processes do and they begin building up the necessary resources we need to survive.

Dr. Porges also stresses the importance of inhibiting our natural defense mechanism to obtain social engagement. To this, we must learn to assess risk, and if we determine a threat is not there, we must actively overpower our natural defense mechanisms. In order to fully develop social engagement responses, we must first understand our emotions, our fears, and our environment. This is why it is our most evolved response state.

The idea of neuroception illustrates why infants are more comfortable around certain people. An infant in his parents' arms will be relaxed and calm. They will even be joyful because they recognize the person and their touch. When the safe infant is in the arms of someone else, they become terrified. They cry out and let people know they don't feel safe. Chemical and biological processes inside of them give the innate ability to recognize an unfamiliar person. Infants may understand far more than we realize.

There are many complicated ways the brain and nervous system, in general, can detect and assess safety concerns. Once we can do this, we are fully developed into our last phase of the hierarchy.

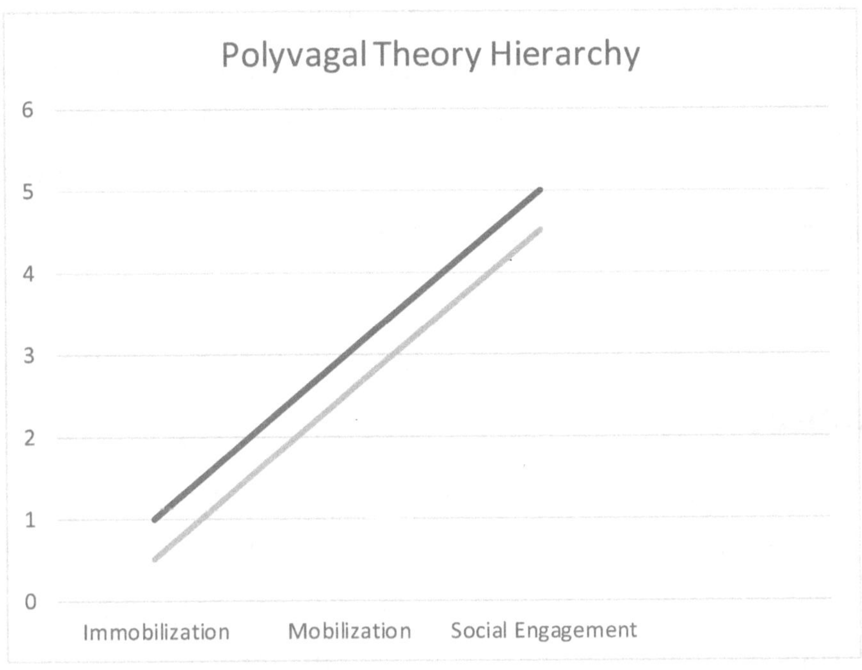

This chart simply represents our progress from immobilization in our early development to social engagement, where we are now. The top line in black showcases this upward moving evolution. The lower gray line represents our ability to cope and handle life issues in general. As we can see, they are quite parallel.

Five States Of The Autonomic Nervous System

For this section, we will get more in-depth into the various advancements of our response system. We will discuss the five states of the autonomic nervous system as it relates to trauma and the associated response. As you will see, these states carry a high fluctuation of emotional responses.

State Zero

This is the initial state of trauma response, which essentially, is before any trauma actually occurs. You are relaxed, breathing and heart rate are normal for you. Your autonomic nervous system is calm but ready to start responding if needed. There is nothing too exciting going on at this state of the autonomic nervous system. This state can be equivalent to social engagement.

State One

This is a mild stress state. You may have increased energy, fear, excitement, irritability, fast thoughts, nervousness, muscles tension, and alertness. This is the initial state of the fight or flight response. Nothing has happened yet, but your senses tell you there is an impending threat. For example, you are walking down an unfamiliar road in the dark. You will be on high-alert and ready to respond as needed.

State Two

This is a high-stress state. You are now in full fight or flight mode. Your heart is racing, you are panicking, your thoughts are moving quickly, you may be hyperventilating, and your muscles are fully contracted. There is a real threat not to your safety and you are ready for action. This basically means fighting for your life or running as fast as you can. State two would occur if you were walking down an unfamiliar road and now you are face to face with an attacker and they are coming for you.

State Three

This is a moderate trauma state. During state 2, you fought, you ran, you used all of your resources to escape physical harm. It did not work, and now you are losing energy. This state is marked by lethargy, sleepiness, hopelessness, slow thoughts, and lessening muscle tension. Your body is getting out of the fight or flight, or mobilization response and slowly transitioning into immobilization. You were trying to fight off your attacker on the unfamiliar road; however, at this moment, you are done fighting and succumb to the threat.

State Four

This is a severe trauma state. You are completely done fighting because all of your resources are exhausted. You will feel disconnected, numb, and just have a blank expression. You are now in full immobilization mode.

These five states breakdown further the hierarchy of polyvagal responses. You may have witnessed or been a victim that went through these various stages. Once you are in-state four, there is no way of going back to state zero, without first passing states one, two, and three.

State Zero→State One→State Two→State Three

State Three→State Two→State One→State Zero

The Basic Exercise

We will be getting into many in-depth exercises about triggering and stimulating the vagus nerve, which in turn will stimulate the autonomic nervous system and affect many different body processes. At this time, we will be talking about the basic exercise for engaging the social engagement response. We will go step by step on how to perform the techniques.

- Lie comfortably on your back, lace the fingers of both hands together, and place them behind your head.

- Rest your head comfortably on your woven fingers. You should feel the hardness of your cranium and also feel the bones of your fingers on your head.

- Keeping your head in one place, look to the right by only moving your eyes. Move them as far as you comfortably can and just keep looking in this direction.

- After a short time, you will either swallow, yawn, or sigh. This is the response that you want. This is a sign of the relaxation of your autonomic nervous system.

- Keep your head still, and bring your eyes back to the center.

- Now, do the same exercise by looking to your left.

- Once you swallow, yawn, or sigh. Relax, and sit up slowly.

- Evaluate how you are feeling at this moment. Are you feeling more relaxed? Has your breathing changed?

The reason we move our eyeballs is that there is a direct connection between the suboccipital muscles and the muscles that move the eyeballs. Also, we do not move our heads is because the rotation of cervical spine 1 and 2 have evolutionary survival value. It can reduce the blood flow to the brain stem, which affects the nerves needed for social engagement. This mechanism is in place so that we can shut off our higher-level responses to go into fight or flight survival mode. The name of this exercise is quite fitting.

Neurofascial Release Technique

The neurofascial release technique is much more like detective work than the basic exercise. If the basic exercise cannot be utilized because the patient may not have the capability of performing it themselves, such as infants or those with developmental disabilities, then the neurofascial release technique will work by detecting strain patterns in the fascia, which is a major connective tissue throughout our body. A light touch is made to the body to help itself identify the issue, and make its corrections by focusing on the touched area. This technique will often cause relief of the fascial strain and normal physiological function will resume.

Chapter 3: Testing The Vagus Nerve

Testing the vagus nerve means to assess its viability and functionality. We can do this through many different processes. For example, when a doctor sticks a tongue depressor in your mouth and tests your gag reflex, he is essentially testing your vagus nerve as well. During the testing process, if problems arise, then we need to find ways to stimulate the vagus nerve and hopefully get it functioning again to its full capacity. In many cases, all we need to do is increase the vagal tone, which means strengthening the vagus nerve and its ability to create a positive influence. Unfortunately, when the vagus nerve is severely damaged, no amount of stimulation will bring it back. We will break this section up by discussing the different methods to test the different portions of the vagus nerve.

Testing the Vagal Function

Back in 1988, Dr. Stephen Porges, along with alternative medicine practitioners John Cottingham and Todd Lyon, published a research project that demonstrated the power of the autonomic nervous system. Through their studies, they determined that the greatest indicator of success when dealing with hands-on therapy sessions the capabilities of the autonomic nervous system. This means that how healthy our autonomic nervous system far exceeds the significance of age, gender, race, or other factors. With their research, they determined that people of all backgrounds could perform well physically if they just had this one area of their bodies taken care of.

During a rolfing technique known as the pelvic lift, Porges, Cottingham, and Lyon gathered several men of varying ages and attached monitors that could assess vagal tone through heart rate variability. When Cottingham performed the test, he could not see the results of the variability in real-time, so his judgment would not be skewed by his prejudices. When it was all said and done, several of the subject who performed well on the test were quite young, with a few being old. They may have concluded that age played the main factor in therapy performance when they just peeked at the surface. However, when they looked deeper into the heart rate variability results, they found that the subjects who performed better had a higher heart rate variability, which is an indicator of vagal tone and autonomic nervous system health.

Through their research, Dr. Porges, Cottingham, and Lyon found that healthy vagal function resulted in better therapy performances. Furthermore, vagal tone plays a major role in heart health, and a person's ability to function daily. This is why we will continually emphasize the importance of the vagus nerve.

Testing The Pharyngeal Branch

The ventral vagus nerve has several branches. One of them is the pharyngeal branch, which innervates the section of the throat immediately behind the nasal cavity and mouth. This is right above the esophagus and larynx. The nerve fibers also go towards the soft palate and the pharynx. So it controls a large portion of the upper throat and oral cavity. This branch of the nerve is responsible for swallowing and vocalizing.

To test this branch, have a person sit straight up in a chair. Have them open their mouth so you can look at the very back of their throats. You should see a bulb-like structure with soft tissue arches on each side. This is the soft palate area. If the person's tongue is in the way, have them hold it down with two fingers. You can also use a tongue depressor, however, be careful to not elicit a gag reflex. You may also use a flashlight or the light on your smartphone for better viewing. When you look inside, the bulb structure and two arches should rise evenly. If they do, this indicates a healthy vagus nerve. If they don't, there may be some dysfunction with the pharyngeal ventral branch. Further assessment and follow up is necessary.

The Gag Reflex

Have you ever tasted something that was not pleasurable or accidentally put something in your mouth the wrong way? If you did, you probably almost threw up or gagged. This is the gag reflex and it showcases your vagus nerve at work. You may have had your gag reflex tested at the doctor's office when they touch the back of your throat with a cotton ball or something soft. This is to test your vagus nerve. If you don't have a gag reflex, this could indicate problems with the vagus nerve. Some people naturally have a stronger gag reflex than others.

Assessing Voice Quality

One of the ways we can assess vagus nerve function is by looking at a person's voice quality. While there is no exact test that can be done, listening to a person's voice can help us determine if their vagus nerve is acting up. This may not be definitive, but it can at least give us information. For example, if a person's voice is quite hoarse, then it could indicate a decreased vagal tone and vagus nerve dysfunction. Again, many things affect a person's vocal cords, but we can certainly use this as a guide.

Heart Rate Variability

Heart rate variability looks at the intervals between consecutive heartbeats in milliseconds and determines the variation. Our heart does not tick evenly throughout the day. It actually varies tremendously. HRV is not the same as counting your heartbeat per minute. We are not acutely aware of this change within milliseconds and specialized tools are needed to accurately assess HRV. One of the key points to take away from here is that the time between each consecutive heartbeat is different from beat to beat. It is never completely uniform. An example of when variation occurs is when we inhale and exhale. When we inhale, our HRV decreases, meaning the distance and time between beats is shorter. When we exhale, our HRV increases, meaning the distance between beats becomes longer. HRV also increases with exercises and other strenuous activities.

The main thing to understand is that the higher a person's HRV, the healthier their autonomic nervous system is. This is because a higher HRV indicates more resiliency and flexibility in the function of the heart. The heart is able to adjust more quickly when it has a higher HRV in general and this allows it to respond to the needs of the body. A lower HRV has been shown to correlate with higher levels of illness and morbidity. Try assessing your HRV by counting your pulse and assessing the difference in time between beats from when you inhale and exhale. This will showcase your HRV.

The reason this is important is that many of the exercises we will mention work by increasing our heart rate variability. Increasing our vagal tone immensely improves upon this factor and improves our heart function. Heart rate is directly impacted by the autonomic nervous system, so increasing its ability to control heart rate through a properly functioning vagus nerve is critical.

We discussed various ways to test the vagus nerve function in this chapter. We also mentioned the study conducted by Dr. Stephen Porges. An objective way you can test your vagus nerve is by assessing your heart rate variability. One way is by counting the variation in beats during different portions of breathing. Also, you may check your HRV when you exercise to see how much it increases from your resting state. HRV is a good self-assessment in determining the health of the vagus nerve.

Chapter 4: Stimulating The Vagus Nerve

When we stimulate the vagus nerve, we unleash its full potential. When we do this, it creates an immense amount of health benefits for ourselves. We will get into the specific Healing Powers in the next chapter. For now, we will discuss several methods that will revitalize and strengthen the vagus nerve. We have discussed the number of functions this vital nerve controls. When utilized properly, it can alter our health in many positive ways. Fo this chapter, we will discuss many specific ways to stimulate the different portions of the vagus nerve.

Yoga, Breathing, Taichi, And Singing

Yoga and taichi are exercises that are powerful for both the body and mind. Not only that, but they are also significant in increasing vagal tone by stimulating the vagus nerve. You will notice a major change in your physical capabilities and your overall mood once you start incorporating these practices into your life.

Yoga

In yoga, conscious deep breathing is a major part of the routine. These deep breaths can target the vagus nerve by inhaling deeply and sucking in our abdominal muscles. It is believed that these abdominal muscles can target the vagus nerve ending where it terminates in the digestive tract. The best way to perform conscious deep breaths is to sit in a peaceful area with your back and neck straight. Good posture is important. Now, slowly breathe in for about 10 seconds and focus on sucking in your abdomen. This will target the vagus nerve. Hold your breath for about 10 seconds if you can, then exhale over about five seconds. Do this about 10 times over several times per day. You will be amazed just how much a few seconds of deep breathing can change your mindset and calm you down.

You can target the vagus nerve in your face my performing a half-smile during your techniques. Imagine yourself half-smiling and hold this position throughout your entire routine. Imagine your jaw softening and a relaxing feeling coming over your head, face, and neck. Dr. Stephen Porges believes that this exercise helps with your social engagement, the most evolved branch of the vagus nerve.

You can help stimulate your vagus nerve by performing yoga postures that open up your chest and throat. This can help stimulate the vagus nerve in your thorax. Start by sitting or kneeling upright, bring your hands to your shoulders and push your elbows together. Inhale as you spread your elbows apart and open up your chest. Exhale as you contract your chest and bring your elbows together. Focus on your inhalation during this technique and do not rush it. This technique is known as "Open your heart".

Releasing the belly is another effective practice for stimulating the vagus nerve through your abdomen. First, put yourself into a table position with your hands underneath your shoulders and your knees underneath your hips. You may place pillows under your knees for more comfort. As you inhale, begin to lift your head and hips while lowering your belly towards the floor. Hold this pose for a few seconds, and then exhale while bringing your head and hips down and pulling your belly up. Imagine a cat when they are stretching and that is the pose you want to mimic. Perform this routine several times, making sure not to overexert yourself. The key is to put thought into breathing and posing.

Many routines in yoga will help stimulate the vagus nerve. We mentioned a few here. Incorporating yoga into your life can have tremendous benefits for your mental and physical health. Lucky for us, there seems to be a yoga studio on every street corner these days and you can also learn routines through online courses.

Tai Chi

Tai chi is another slow-paced, low impact exercise that can significantly increase our vagal tone. The intention of tai chi is slow deep breathing and having the ability to relax. This is the moment where the body has time to regenerate. Like yoga, tai chi techniques utilize various breathing, stretching and posing techniques. Many of them target the vagus nerve, which effectively stimulates it. The techniques of tai chi require a person to stand still for long periods with focus and concentration. During this time, they also focus on various deep breathing exercises that create a sense of relaxation throughout the body, which will actively stimulate the vagus nerve. Continuous activation of the vagus nerve will help to keep a strong vagal tone. Just like with yoga, take the time to learn proper tai chi practices through a properly trained instructor or course.

Singing

Do you love to sing to yourself, whether in the shower, driving in your car, or just sitting at home alone? It probably makes you feel quite good and uplifts your mood. There may be more benefits to this than you think. Since your vagus nerve is connected to your vocal cords, a healthy dose of singing can immensely stimulate the vagus nerve. The vibration from singing, gargling, and chanting can all contribute to increasing vagal tone.

Kundalini Breath Of Fire

The purpose of Kundalini yoga is to awaken the kundalini energy at the base of the spine. There are two lines of kundalini energy that target the various chakras, or energy focal points in our body. These chakras, when released, have various health benefits depending on the particular one. There are believed to be seven chakras that surround the spinal column. Kundalini is thought to be a life force that travels up the entire spine up to the pineal gland, which it fires up. Once the energy begins flowing through the body, the yoga practitioner becomes more aware and integrated with reality, and they move into a higher state of consciousness. This essentially leads to a happier, more productive, and more fulfilling life.

The breath of fire is a breathing technique in the art of yoga that places an equal emphasis on inhaling and exhaling. The navel point is sucked in towards the spine on exhalation, and released out during inhalation. Also, the breathing is done through the nostrils while the eyes and mouth are closed. Once a person starts doing these exercises, they are meant to begin feeling better shortly after.

The Kundalini energy has often been depicted symbolically as a serpent that coils around the base of the spinal column. This represents the energy that also wraps itself around the spine. Also, the serpent has been used to symbolize rebirth and rejuvenation because of its ability to shed its old skin. The kundalini energy is also believed to bring about rejuvenation and rebirth in people.

Kundalini And The Vagus Nerve

There is believed to be great synergy between the kundalini energy and the vagus nerve. Kundalini energy brings information back to the brain and follows much of the same path as the vagus nerve. Many yogis believe they are very well connected for this reason. Many practitioners of kundalini yoga have even equated the vagus nerve to the kundalini serpent.

The vagus nerve is believed to be a major life force in the practice of yoga. Here are a few similarities between the vagus nerve and kundalini:

- The vagus nerve is two nerves recognized as one. The kundalini is two separate energy channels that function as one when they become purified.

- The vagus nerve runs from the colon to the brain. The kundalini rests in the first chakra at the base of the spine in the pelvic floor and rises to the pineal gland at the center of the brain.

- Vagus nerve and kundalini both run through the spinal cord.

- They both touch and interact with the organs along the spine.

- The vagus nerve takes information from the stomach and dysfunctions in the vagus nerve can lead to stomach problems. The kundalini has a main psychic center in the navel. When this center is not activated, the stomach and digestive can result due to disempowerment.

- The heart directly communicates with the brain through the vagus nerve. The heart chakra and pineal gland interact with each other through the kundalini energy life-force.

Because of the many similarities, practitioners of kundalini yoga believe that the vagus nerve is simply a physical manifestation of the kundalini life force. When the vagus nerve is opened up, just like the kundalini, it can manage all of the cosmic energy in the world and universe. If it is unable to do this, then major illnesses and dysfunctions will show up in the body. Within the kundalini mindset, it is believed that the things that bring us joy and peace, are the best ways to increase vagal tone function. We will showcase this idea in a big way during this chapter.

Cold Exposure

Cold exposure has been shown to increase vagus nerve stimulation in a major way. Many high functioning and productive people have found that taking a cold shower in the morning revitalizes them and they feel much more energized throughout the day. Cold exposure has been shown to decrease the sympathetic response, and in turn, increase parasympathetic activity through the vagus nerve.

Begin slowly incorporating cold exposure into your life. This does not have to be an immediate process. Start by turning the water cold for about 30 seconds while you shower. Increase exposure time day by day from there. Also, start wearing fewer layers each time you go out into the cold. Splashing cold water on your face can also be beneficial. Do whatever activities you can think of to increase your exposure to a cold environment.

Valsalva Maneuver

This maneuver is performed by moderately forcing exhalation against a closed airway. You may have used this technique when you were up in an airplane and needed to unclog your ears. Simply cover your nose and mouth and then try to breathe out. This maneuver will increase the pressure in your thorax which will also temporarily increase vagal tone. The

Valsalva maneuver is often employed when trying to reduce a rapid heart rate. When performing this maneuver, it is important to sit down to prevent heart rate and blood pressure from dropping too quickly. This goes back to the vasovagal syncope.

Probiotics

Since there is a direct connection between the gut and the brain, having healthy microbiota in the digestive tract has been shown to increase vagal tone.

Humming

Just like with singing, the vibration from humming can stimulate the vagus nerve near your vocal cords and effectively increase vagal tone. Sit in a quiet place and create a low, steady and continuous sound, similar to a bee.

Laughing And Socializing

Much research suggests that laughing and socializing immensely increases vagal tone. You will also decrease your stress hormones. When you are having a good time, you are doing better for your health than you ever imagined. Next time your friends invite you out, it may benefit you to go with them.

Smiling

Smiling has been shown to also target the vagus nerve. The vagus nerve innervates several areas in the upper throat and near the oral cavity. Smiling regularly can help to stimulate the vagus nerve branches in this area. We mentioned the half-smile during yoga sessions. You can perform these or even a full smile regularly. Smiling, in general, improves your overall mood.

The Salamander Exercise

This exercise is pretty much what it sounds like. You get on the ground and crawl like a salamander. This routine is great for the majority of the muscles in the body and targets your vagus nerve through the core. The following steps will discuss how to do the salamander exercise properly

- Get on the ground and lie on your stomach.

- Rotate your head to your right and reach out with your left arm like your crawling forward. At the same time, pull your right leg under you. Then rotate your head to the left while reaching with your right arm and pulling your left leg under you. Keep switching sides and do this exercise for as long as you can tolerate.

- You can lie in place or move forward during this exercise. Whichever one is easier for you.

- Make sure you are not dragging your limbs but picking them up as you move.

Before doing this exercise, make sure to stretch appropriately. Doing so will help prevent potential injury to various muscle groups. You may also want to put down some padding like a yoga mat. The salamander exercise is almost like swimming on land.

Neck Extension Exercises

When our neck muscles become too tight, it can create pressure on our vagus nerve. When there's pressure with this nerve at the base of the skull, several of its functions below this area are becoming impeded. Since the majority of the vagus nerve lies below the base of the skull, this will create several different issues. Several neck extension exercises can reduce this pressure and open up the pathway for the vagus nerve.

- Neck flexion is an exercise that increases the downward range of motion in your neck and shoulders. To perform, sit down in a chair with your back straight and your feet flat on the floor. Be in as relaxed a position as you can be. Slowly pull your chin down to your chest and hold this position for about 10 seconds before coming back up. Repeat this motion about 10 times, being careful not to strain too much. Do not perform this quickly, but easy on the way up and way down. Make sure you are feeling the stretch and holding the position to get the full effect.

- Neck extension to retraction exercise will stretch out and strengthen the muscles on the side of your neck, shoulders and upper back. Sit down in a chair with your feet flat on the floor and your head extending out beyond your neck. You should feel slight tension in your neck. From this position, draw your head back slowly and bring your chin to your neck. Draw in as far as you can and then hold this position for several seconds. Repeat about 10 times or until you are fatigued.

- Isometric neck extension exercises will help build and relax the muscles in your upper neck and shoulders. Stand up straight with your knees slightly bent and your arms at your sides. Now place your hands behind your neck and have your elbows bent out in front of you. Push your head back against the resistance of your hands and hold for about 10 seconds. Bring your head back to a normal position. Do this about 10 times.

- Basic neck extension exercises will increase the range of motion in the muscles at the back of the neck. This practice will significantly reduce the pressure on your vagus nerve. Sit down in a chair with your back straight, your arms at your side, and your feet on the floor. Tilt your head back until the back portion of your head touches the back portion of your neck. Hold this for about 10 seconds before returning to a normal position. Repeat this about 10 times.

Doing these exercises will relieve pain and tension in all areas of your neck. Besides, they will help to improve vagus nerve function. After doing these exercises regularly, you may begin to see improvements in other areas of your health that are impacted by the vagus nerve. For example, your digestion may improve.

SCM Exercises

Moving further with exercises for a stiff neck, the sternocleidomastoid muscle, or SCM, is a major muscle in the neck that attaches the skull to the sternum and the clavicle bone. The vagus nerve sits right in front of the SCM as it runs down the neck, so dysfunctions in this muscle can heavily affect the crucial nerve. We will discuss several exercises that target the SCM and improve overall health and movement of the muscle. In turn, this can lead to better health and function of the vagus nerve.

- **Side neck and rotation stretch:** This stretch involves rotating the neck and bending it sideways which will lengthen the SCM. Stand straight and perform a neck retraction. Bend your neck to the left while rotating your chin in the opposite direction and upward until you feel the right-side stretch. Hold for about 20 seconds, or until you feel comfortable.

- **Wall side neck bridge:** This involves lateral flexion of the SCM. Stand against the wall with your left side, and also lean your head against it. Hold hands behind your back and move your feet to the right so you are lean diagonally to the left against the wall. Keep your legs straight and feet touching. Next, push against the wall to tilt your body to the left and move your body to the right. Turn around and repeat the exercise on the other side.

- **Wall front neck bridge:** This exercise works through forwarding flexion to strengthen the SCM. Take a small cushioned mat and place it against the wall to the height of your chest. Place your forehead against the mat and step back while keeping your legs straight. Align your back with your legs while also holding your hands behind your back. Move your back and hips forward by carefully extending your chin to the mat. Make sure to use a cushion for this exercise and not a pillow or something that will slip down.

- **Neck retraction:** Align your neck with your whole spine by pulling back your chin. Repeat this about 20 times. This exercise strengthens the SCM and also improves excess forward posture.

Perform these exercises regularly and you will experience noticeable changes in your SCM strength and flexibility in no time. Also, you may begin to notice other health improvements related to vagus nerve health.

Exercises To Improve Posture

The neck pains that we discussed in a previous section can be caused by poor posture. We will also get into the negative health consequences resulting from this in a later chapter. Once you see those, this section will seem much more important to you. You may not realize just how much of an impact the way you stand has on your health, but as far as long term results, it is crucial. For now, we will discuss specific exercises that will improve your posture, and in turn, improve your vagus nerve function and overall health. Take precautions not to strain yourself during these exercises. If you are not a flexible person, it will take time to reach where you need to be. Take it slow and increase your limits daily. Trying to force yourself the first day may cause unnecessary injury and deter you from doing these exercises in the future.

- **Child's pose:** This pose stretches your spine, glutes, and hamstrings. And also helps to release pressure in your lower back and neck.

    o Sit on your shin bones with both of your knees together. Keep your toes connected and your heels spread apart.

- Fold forward at your hips and slowly walk yourself forward using your hands.

    - Sink your hips towards your feet. Gently turn your head to one side. You may also touch the floor with your forehead.

    - Keep your arms extended.

    - Breath deeply, targeting your waist and back of your rib cage.

    - Try to relax and stay in this pose for five minutes, taking deep breaths the whole time.

- **Forward fold:** This simple stretch releases tension in your spine, glutes, and hamstrings. You should feel your entire backside opening up.

    - Stand straight up with your big toes touching and heels slightly spread apart.

    - Bring your hands to your hips and fold forward at this location.

    - Release your hands and reach towards the floor. You don't have to touch the ground. Just go as far down as you can.

- o Bend your knees slightly, soften your hip joints, and allow your spine to lengthen more.

- o Tuck your chin into your chest and hold this pose for about a minute. You should see yourself being able to go further and further each day.

- **Standing cat/cow stretch:** This stretch will help you loosen up your spine, back, hips, and glutes.

  - o Stand so your feet align with your hip and bend your knees slightly.

  - o Extend your hands in front of you or you can place them on your thighs.

  - o Lengthen your neck, bring your chin to your chest, and round out your spine.

  - o Then look up, lift your chest, and move your spine in the opposite direction.

  - o While holding each of the positions, take about five breaths.

  - o Repeat this step for several minutes.

- **High Plank:** This exercise may seem difficult and strenuous at first, but it actually relieves tension throughout your body and strengthens your shoulders, glutes, and hamstrings.

  - Come down on all fours, straighten your legs, raise your hips, and lift your heels.

  - Straighten your back and engage your abdominal, arm, and leg muscles.

  - Lengthen the back of your neck, loosen your throat and look down on the floor.

  - Keep your chest open and your shoulders back.

  - Try to hold this pose for one minute. Of course, the first time you do it will be very difficult. Start with 30 seconds and then build up each day.

- **Side plank:** This pose works on the muscles of your sides and glutes. Strengthening these muscles will play a big role in improving your posture.

  - From the high plank position from before, bring your left hand to the center of your body.

- o Bring all of your weight onto your left hand, stack your feet, and raise your right hip.

- o Extend your right hand towards the ceiling or place on your hips.

- o Maintain this pose while engaging your abdominals, side body, and glutes.

- o Align your body from head to heels in a straight line.

- o If you need more support, you may bring your left knee to the floor.

- o Look straight ahead and hold this pose for 30 seconds.

- o Come back to high plank position and then repeat steps for the other side.

- **Downward facing dog:** This is a forward bend that can be used as a resting pose to balance yourself out. This pose stretches and aligns your back muscles and can also do a lot for improving back pain.

- o Use a yoga mat of some sort and lie with your stomach on the floor. Press into your hands as you tuck your toes under your feet and lift your heels.

- o Lift your knees and hips to bring your sitting bones to the ceiling.

- o Bend your knees slightly to lengthen your spine.

- o Keep your ears in alignment with your upper arms.

- o Press firmly into your hands and keep your heels slightly lifted.

- o Keep this pose for one minute. You may repeat several times as tolerated.

- **Pigeon pose:** This pose opens up your hips and loosens your spine, glutes, and hamstrings. It can also open up the sciatic nerve and quadriceps. Working on all these areas of the body will play a significant role in improving posture.

  - o Come down on all fours with your knees below your hips and your hands slightly out in front of your shoulders.

  - o Move your knee up behind your right wrist and angle your right foot to the left.

o   Rest the outside of your right shin on the floor.

o   Stretch your left leg back by straightening the knee and resting your thigh on the floor.

o   Slowly lower your torso down to rest your inner right thigh with both hands extended out in front of you.

o   Hold this position for about one minute.

o   Release the position by slowly walking your hands back towards your hips and lifting your torso.

o   Repeat these steps using the other side.

- **Thoracic spine rotation:** This exercise relieves tightness and pain in our back.

o   Come down on all fours and sink your hips down towards your heels. Rest them on your shins.

o   Place your left hand behind your head with your elbow extended to the side.

o   Keep your right hand under your shoulder.

- Exhale as you lift your left elbow towards the ceiling. This will stretch the front of your torso.

  - Take one long inhale and then exhale in this position.

  - Release and go back down to your original position.

  - Repeat this position about five to 10 times and in both directions.

- **Glute Squeezes:** This exercise works to strengthen your glutes and relieve lower back pain. It will also work on the alignment of your hips and pelvis, leading to a much better posture.

  - Lie on your back with your knees bent and your feet spread at about the width of your hips.

  - Keep your feet about a foot away from your hips.

  - Rest your arms on the side of your body with your palms facing down.

  - Exhale as you bring your feet closer to your hips.

  - Hold this position for about 10 seconds and then slowly move your feet further away.

o   Do this exercise about 10 times.

Many exercises can improve your posture. If you are a fan of yoga, then you probably noticed a few familiar poses. We mentioned yoga earlier as a way to stimulate the vagus nerve. Yoga is also great at relieving neck and back pain and improving posture. This will, in turn, further help the vagus nerve.

The biggest issue with posture is that we don't realize we have it throughout the day. Most of us are not conscious of keeping our back and neck straight as we are moving around. We are doing a lot of strenuous work which puts a strain on most of our body parts. Start paying attention to your posture. Walk and also sit in proper positions. Be aware of your body mechanics too. Finally, perform the previous exercises regularly to maintain strong and flexible back muscles and other supporting structures that relate to our posture. Don't ignore neck and back pain either. It may just be a mere nuisance right now but in the long run, it can have drastic results for the vagus nerve and our overall health.

Trapezius Muscle's Twisting And Turning Exercises

The Trapezius muscle is one of the widest muscles of the back. They cover the back, neck, and upper trunk area. The major muscle links the back portion of the vertebrae to the spine, scapulae (shoulder blades), ribs, and clavicle. The trapezius is very close to the surface of the skin. The vagus nerve runs in close quarters with the spinal accessory nerve, which feeds the trapezius muscle. Strengthening the trapezius muscle can have a direct impact on both nerves. In addition, since the trapezius muscle is a major muscle in the back, it can play a role in forwarding head posture too. We will go twist and turn exercises that can improve the tone of the muscles, improve breathing, lengthen the spine and alleviate back and neck pain. The goal is not so much to strengthen the muscles, as it is already pretty strong. It is more to wake them up so they can share the workload. We often ignore the trapezius muscle without realizing it, especially when our posture becomes poor. Here are the steps:

- Sit comfortably on a firm surface, such as a chair or bench, and keep your face looking forward.

- Fold and cross your arms with your hands resting gently on your elbows.

- You will be rotating your shoulder girdle from side to side briskly without stopping. Do not move your hips or lower back.

- For the first part, let your elbows drop and rest in front of your body. Rotate only your shoulders so your elbows move from side to side. Allow your arms to glide gently over your stomach. This activates the fibers of your upper trapezius.

After doing this exercise several times, you will notice that your head feels lighter and your neck has more mobility. If someone were to look at you from the side, they would notice your head protruding less forward than before.

Positive Self-Talk With Guided Imagery

It seems that everyone is touting positivity these days. A positive mind will lead to a positive life that seems to be the mantra of many people. However, just because it's commonplace to say, does not mean that it is not effective. Positive self-talk has been shown to uplift a person's spirits and reduces their anxiety in the process. This reduction in anxiety helps to calm the nervous system and has been shown to increase vagal tone. Since this is a case, there is a major physiological benefit to being positive. There is no real rule about how to talk positively to yourself. In general, tell yourself what you need to improve your mindset.

With this technique, you actually don't even need to speak with words. You can also have positive thoughts. Many people use positive imagery. They think about something that brings them joy, comfort, and excitement. This can be an area, person, goal, or any other image. The key is that it brings you some calmness and you begin to feel good about yourself and your life. Do not dismiss the idea of positivity. It may not solve all of your problems, but it can change your mindset and allow you to handle life in a better way.

EFT Meridian Tapping

The concepts of EFT Meridian Tapping are similar to those of acupuncture. EFT stands for emotional freedom technique and is an alternative method to reduce physical pain and emotional distress. Meridian points are certain spots that can be mapped out throughout the body. Energy circulates throughout these network channels and can be tapped into at any of these specific points. Physical and emotional issues are a result of disruptions in the energy fields of the body. Tapping restores the energy balance and negative emotions are conquered.

The technique works by first focusing on a negative emotion that you are having. This can be fear, anxiety, hate, sadness, or any number of emotions. While focusing on this mental issue that is bothering you, use your fingertips to tap on any one of the meridians points five to seven times. Tapping on these points will access your body's energy, restoring it to a balanced state.

The nine meridian points in the body are:

- The heel of your hand

- Eyebrows

- Below your eyes

- Side of your eye

- Under your nose

- Under your chin

- below your collar bone

- Under your arm

- On top of your head

Each meridian point's energy is attached to a specific organ, so when you are tapping the particular spot, you are accessing that particular organ. For example, the spot on the heel of your hand corresponds to the small intestine.

Rezzimax Tuning Device

The Rezzimax tuning device is a portable tuner that combines resonance with various stress management techniques. Using this device properly will help manage and alleviate neck pain, headaches, and TMJ pain. The tuner will also target the vagus nerve, stimulating it through proper positioning and vibrations. Various exercises can be performed that will help harness the power of the vagus nerve. First of all, place the tuner probes on the sides of the neck. The tuner is shaped like a clip. Clip it on the neck muscles from behind and use a pillow to position properly. Allow the tuning device to vibrate for 30-60 seconds.

There are a few more positions you can use. Place the probe on the top portion of the head near the front. Allow it to vibrate for 30-60 seconds. Next, place the probes on the temples, also allowing to vibrate for 30-60 seconds. Finally, place the probes on the bridge of the nose and repeat one more time. Targeting these specific locations when using the device will aim the vagus nerve and provide direct stimulation.

The Rezzimax tuning device will provide a combination of stimulating your vagus nerve and improving your pain without the aid of many pharmaceuticals. We aim to show you ways to heal your body using your own body processes and this device will go a long way in doing so.

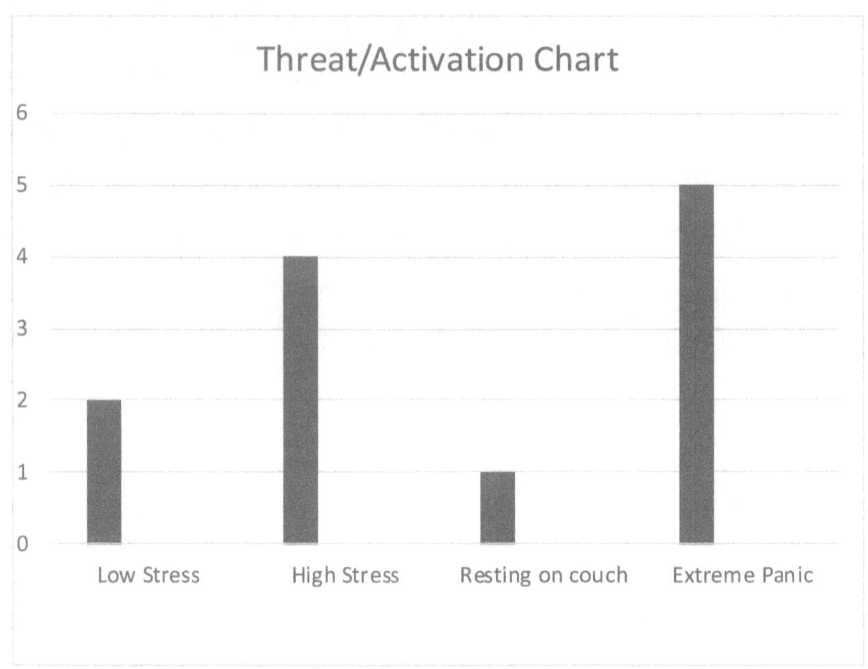

This bar graph illustrates the relationship between threat and activation. The key on the bottom shows the threat and stress levels and the height of the graph showcases the amount of activation with each level.

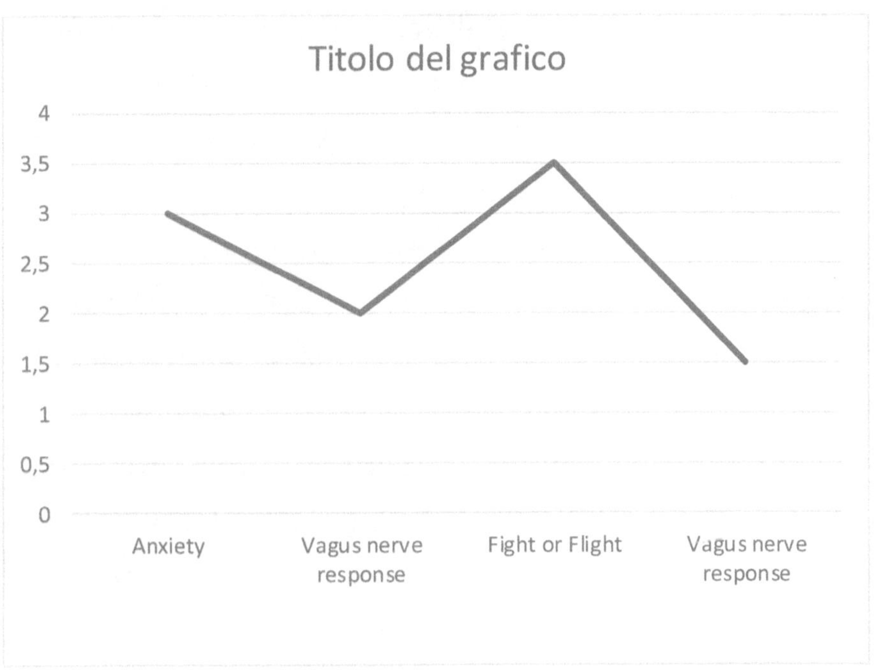

This line graph showcases how vagus nerve stimulation and response can reduce high alertness and bring us to a more calming state from various other responses.

A Real Example

We have gone over many examples of how to stimulate the vagus nerve. We want to provide a real-life example of how it has saved someone in an emergency. Many of the techniques we discussed above can be used at a moment's notice, like deep breathing and the Valsalva maneuver.

During a flight on a major airline, a passenger began feeling quite sick. He did not know what was going on, but he could feel his chest pounding. When he felt his pulse, it was too fast to even count, but he knew it was going well over 100 beats per minute. He was panicking for sure; however, based on his experience as a healthcare worker, he remembered the Valsalva maneuver to initiate the vasovagal response. He performed this technique while also baring down like he was to have a bowel movement. He performed this several times and could feel his heart rate coming down slowly. When he rechecked his pulse, it back in the 80s. He also felt much better and did not draw too much attention to himself.

A few times during the flight, he would perform the Valsalva maneuver again just to be safe. He also realized he was dehydrated and drank some extra water. This helped him get through the rest of the flight.

This particular maneuver helped the passenger initiate the vasovagal response quickly, which significantly reduced his heart rate to sustainable levels. If he had not done that, he likely would have passed out or worse. This is a major example of how stimulating the vagus nerve actually saved someone's life at the moment.

Chapter 5: Healing Powers Of The Vagus Nerve

In what ways can the vagus nerve heal us? That is what we will discuss here. The vagus nerve literally can have superpowers when it is used to its full potential. From long-term physical illnesses to major mood disorders, the vagus nerve has the potential to help us in ways we could never imagine. After we go over the multitude of diseases that can be improved and even avoided by using the healing powers of the vagus nerve, the practices to test and stimulate this powerful structure will become much more obvious. We will break this chapter down into the specific mental and physical ailments that can be healed.

Migraines And Headaches

Many people around the world experience migraines and headaches. For some, they occur on an isolated basis, while others deal with them chronically. Furthermore, for some, they are a simple nuisance, but for others, they become debilitating. While there is no known cause of migraines, it is believed to be due to abnormal activity in the brain. Many of the triggers are related to stress and overactivity. That being said, finding ways to relax the body and mind can certainly have positive impacts on reducing painful and consistent headaches. A common method of treating these disorders is through simple medications, like over the counter pain pharmaceuticals, or more aggressive medications for severe cases. People have even had expensive procedures and tests done to rid themselves of chronic migraines and headaches.

Much research has been done regarding the effects of vagus nerve stimulation and the prevention of major headaches. While the science is still out in many ways about how this occurs, many researchers feel that the interconnectivity of the vagus nerve and other cranial nerves plays a major role in improving these painful disorders. Improving migraines and headaches was not an initial goal of stimulation. Scientists and medical professionals were studying various other ways stimulation could impact the body, like with epilepsy, and through this, many of the subjects involved reported a marked improvement in their headaches.

It is fair to say that conducting the various number of activities to stimulate the vagus nerve can help to heal people with excessive and even debilitating migraines and headaches. If simple exercises that you can do at home will improve your quality of life, then they are worth giving a try. Also, if they are just as, or more effective than putting a foreign substance in your body, that these practices become even more beneficial.

Massage And Migraines

Stimulating it in any way can help to increase vagal tone, effectively increasing relaxation throughout the body. Massage helps to rclax the muscles and the body as a whole. Massage therapy has shown to increase vagal tone and effectively decrease long-term migraines.

There are specific massage techniques that can be done that specifically target the vagus nerve. Some examples include deep abdominal massages where the vagus nerve ends, as well as on the sides of the neck where the carotid artery runs. The vagus nerve runs alongside the carotid artery. If you can pinpoint these various locations and massage them properly, then they can be very effective in reducing migraines. It is recommended that you seek out a highly trained professional to perform these massages on you to prevent serious injuries.

Fibromyalgia

Widespread musculoskeletal pain coupled with sleep issues, fatigue, mood problems, and poor memory is all characterized by this disorder. Researchers believe that how our brain processes pain is altered, which amplifies the sensation of pain. Also, it is believed that repeated nerve stimulation changes a person's brain chemistry, causing a heightened reaction to pain.

During a major study in 2011, researchers found that a significant number of participants reported decreased pain and tenderness after vagus nerve stimulation. While they admitted much more research needs to be done, they were definitely impressed with the initial findings. Once again, it is not fully known how vagus nerve stimulation reduces fibromyalgia pain; it is believed that the reduction in nerve stimulation by increasing vagal tone plays a big part in this. When this powerful nerve is stimulated, it allows the nerves, muscles, and other tissues in our body that are related to the pain to slow down and relax. In this manner, vagus nerve stimulation can effectively heal fibromyalgia pain. Of course, there is no known cure for this disorder at the moment, but more research on the vagus nerve may just change that.

Tachycardia

Tachycardia is when your heart is beating at an increased rate, generally above 100. Tachycardia is usually a result of another issue like heart disease, kidney failure, or dehydration. In addition, an increased heart rate is a natural response to things like stress or exercise. Whatever the cause, your heart is beating faster than the normal limits.

The vagus nerve mediates the parasympathetic innervation of the heart. The nerve specifically affects the sinoatrial node, which is the heart's internal pacemaker. Increasing vagal tone through stimulation will reduce the heart rate significantly as it increases the relaxation response. Next time you feel your heart rate speed up, try doing some deep breathing exercises and see how much your heart rate slows down. Again, take proper precautions to not overstimulate your vagus nerve.

As a side note, the vagus nerve will also decrease a person's blood pressure. Increasing our vagal tone through stimulation will decrease blood pressure in the same manner as heart rate by engaging the parasympathetic nervous system.

Problems With Poor Posture

Poor posture, especially long-term, can have more detrimental effects than we realize. If you are always slouching forward, remember that you are creating long-term health problems for yourself that goes beyond physical limitations. You can impact your vital organs and tissues and may end up dealing with many longterm illnesses. Here are several ways that posture can impact our health.

- The most obvious issues are musculoskeletal problems. When your posture is not balanced, and you are constantly slouching forward, this will put extra pressure on certain vertebrate in your back and neck. This can eventually lead to damaging the ligaments and discs in this area. Also, by leaning forward, the muscles in the front become tight, while the muscles in the back become strained. Any extra activity and stress can lead to further injury. Of course, mobility will be reduced, the pain will increase, and our overall quality of life will be reduced.

- Poor posture equals poor breathing. Slouching causes your thorax to become compressed, which leads to your lungs not being able to expand normally. Your diaphragm will also not be able to move properly.

Excessive compression of the chest and diaphragm will also lead to vagus nerve dysfunction as the vagal tone will decrease due to the body becoming more stationary over time. Remember that the vagus has to be stimulated through movement for it to function properly.

- Poor posture can also lead to poor digestion. This may be a little difficult to understand. Yes, slouching can also compress the abdominal cavity, which can affect digestion. However, there is a more complex reason why digestion is reduced. When we slouch and pull our shoulders forward, we still need to be able to see. As a natural reaction, we will tilt our heads back. Doing this can compress the vagus nerve at the base of the skull, which will reduce its functionality. For us to have proper digestion, we must have a properly functioning vagus nerve.

We discussed several exercises that will improve our posture, and also the viability of our vagus nerve. If you find yourself slouching, start doing these exercises to see if you can improve your stance. Now that we know the long-term effects of having poor posture, we must work to improve it.

Vagus Nerve And Anxiety

Anxiety refers to the experience of fear or apprehension in response to something that is about to happen or may happen in the future. This can be a dangerous situation or having to take an exam. It is created by a sense of uncertainty about our environment or ourselves. A small amount of anxiety is commonplace during stress. It can often work as a defense mechanism to keep us alert and aware. However, when anxiety gets out of hand, it can become debilitating. We spoke earlier about immobilization and mobilization responses according to Dr. Stephen Porges. This is a perfect example. Initially, anxiety can trigger us to get moving and overcome whatever is creating the fear in us. However, when the anxiety becomes overwhelming, we freeze up and go into the immobilization phase.

Since anxiety heightens all of our physiological responses, stimulating the vagus nerve can lower these responses. For example, when you are feeling overly anxious, try to find a quiet place and take some deep, conscious breaths. After a while, you will feel your body calm down as well as your anxiety.

Vagus Nerve And Depression

Depression is a mood disorder marked by extreme feelings of sadness. While feeling sad alone is not depression, it is a major symptom. People often feel hopeless and useless. Depression can be short-term and related to a major life event. However, in some cases, it becomes a chronic illness with severe mental and physical health consequences.

Vagus nerve stimulation has been shown to decrease feelings of depression over time. The reason is not known; however, researchers feel it is due to the changing of the wave patterns in the brain. Doing several of the exercises we mentioned above may do wonders for getting you out of your depressive mood.

Autism Spectrum Disorders

Autism is a complex neurobehavioral disorder. It is characterized by poor reciprocal social interaction, impairment in communication, and the presence of repetitive patterns of behavior, interests, and activities. Children typically begin having symptoms very early in their development, generally before age three. The level of the impairment determines exactly where on the spectrum a person falls. Some people are very low on the spectrum and still fully capable of living relatively normal lives, while others are very high on the spectrum and will never be fully functional.

Autism And The Role Of Hearing

Hearing loss can often be a precursor to autism spectrum disorder. The Gallaudet Institute estimates that 1 in 59 kids who have hearing loss also have autism. Often, early signs of autism may mimic hearing disorders. Understanding the various signs of autism is important, especially in young children. Some of these include:

- Lack or delay in the spoken language

- Lack of interest in social engagement

- Lack of eye contact

- Repetitive use of language and other mannerisms

- Lack of imagination, which includes make-believe play

- Fixation on specific parts of objects.

Some children with autism will have no hearing loss; others will have it on some level. Many children who experience hearing disorders will have other developmental issues as well, including autism spectrum disorder. A child with autism may also process sounds differently, even if their hearing is normal. In these cases, they will have trouble with learning and language. Things can become quite complicated with children who have autism because their hearing may be hypersensitive in certain cases, while they may appear to have hearing loss in other cases. For example, they will be extremely sensitive to high-pitched sounds, but can't pick up on low-pitched sounds. An audiologist or speech pathologist may be able to help a child by providing hearing aids, speech and communication training, computer-based tools and a wealth of other techniques.

We discussed some of the signs of autism. The following are some of the signs of a hearing disorder with no signs of autism.

- Uses eyes to watch people

- Enjoys hugs

- Sometimes socially isolated due to not being able to communicate well

- Accepts changes rather than being repetitive (autistic children will often be very resistant to change)

With many tests being available to test hearing, disorders of this type are being diagnosed earlier. In many cases, it can be detected after an infant is born and before they leave the hospital. Hearing and other developmental disorders may also clue us into potential autism spectrum disorders.

Vagus Nerve And Autism

Some new scientific studies suggest that the vagus nerve may contribute to autism. The findings are still quite preliminary; however, researchers have found that some children with autism have slower development in their respiratory sinus arrhythmia or RSA. RSA is basically the fluctuations in heart rate when inhaling versus exhaling. The heart rate speeds up when we inhale and slows down when we exhale. This is controlled by the vagus nerve. Several previous studies have shown that RSA is less pronounced in children with autism than in children without autism. It is unknown whether insufficient RSA causes autism or is a result of autism. It is a very interesting theory to think about, though.

Many researchers are also determining whether vagus nerve stimulation can lead to an improvement in hearing disorders in those who live with autism. Some studies on rodents have suggested the ability to distinguish sounds improved with increasing vagal tone. The findings are also preliminary but may suggest similar results in humans.

Technique For Rounding The Flat Back Of The Head

Flathead syndrome is when a flat spot develops on the back of a baby's head. This is also known as plagiocephaly. An infant's skull bones do not fully fuse together until they are several months only, so their head is quite pliable. These flat spots are often caused by sleeping in the same position for long periods. Infants should sleep on their backs, but while they are awake, they need to lie on their tummies too, so they avoid these flats post on their heads.

If you notice an infant with a flat spot on their head, it is important to consult a specialist for advice or interventions. There is a technique used for rounding out the flat back of the head. The steps are as follows:

- Start by feeling the two Sternocleidomastoid muscles on each side, and work on the tighter one.

- Take the top of the SCM muscle gently and firmly between the thumb and index finger. Careful not to cause pain.

- Ask someone to hold the foot on the side where we will release the SCM.

- Gently bend the child's foot at the ankle joint with one hand, and then gently bend the toes up with the other hand.

- After a minute or two, the child relaxes and so does the SCM.

- When the SCM no longer pulls on one side of the cranium, the flat spot slowly fills out and becomes rounded.

- The two sides will now be symmetrical.

Generally, beyond this technique, the flat head syndrome does not need any other medical interventions as long as it is not congenital. With congenital plagiocephaly, where the sutures in between the skull bones close prematurely, further intervention may be needed. However, even when it's congenital, it is more of a cosmetic issue than medical. It usually does not affect brain development. Otherwise, be mindful of your baby's sleeping position and rotate regularly. In some cases, there are molding helmets available that can help reshape an infant's head to be symmetrical.

Vagus Nerve And PTSD

PTSD, Post-traumatic stress disorder, is caused by major trauma and creates major psychological disorders. It is often most associated with military personnel; however, it can also be common for first-responders, healthcare workers, police officers, and just about anybody that has gone through a major traumatic event. Individuals with PTSD may suffer from anxiety, depression, intrusive memories, negative thoughts, and chronic pain.

Several of the therapies we discussed prior will help to stimulate the vagus nerve, and particularly the ventral vagal portions, which deals with positivity and social engagement. When we can target this area of the nerve, then we can help people heal from past trauma. With PTSD, it is very important to remember the polyvagal theory of Dr. Porges and the hierarchy of development. We must understand what response phase a person is in before we proceed to help them. If they are in the most primitive phase of immobilization, then we must move them into mobilization for a short-term period, before we transition to social engagement.

Let's use the example of someone who went through sexual assault. We will say that her experience was so mortifying, that she eventually became closed off to the world and has no ability in her present state to make any changes in her life. She is suffering from major PTSD due to what occurred. At first, she may have gone into the fight or flight response; however, after being overpowered for so long, she eventually had to give up the fight. This caused her to lie down and become immobilized. The key now is to work on several mind and body techniques to wake her up and push her into a mobilization mindset. Once she is in the mobilization phase, then she can fight and move forward. She can become active and start taking steps to get past her trauma. Eventually, with the proper path and techniques, she will become socially engaged and start trusting again.

Vagus Nerve And Bipolar Disorder

Bipolar disorder is a mental illness marked by extreme mood changes that go from high to low and vice versa. A person may be manic one minute and depressed the next. The changes in mood may even be mixed. Signs of bipolar disorder can be divided into two groups: mania and depression.

Mania

- Feeling excessively happy for long periods

- Not needing much sleep

- Feeling restless or impulsive

- Talking very fast with racing thoughts

- Being very overconfident in one's abilities

- Having no concentration and getting distracted easily

- Taking unnecessary risks like gambling with life savings

Depression

- Feelings of sadness and hopelessness that won't go away

- Withdrawing from loved ones

- Major appetite changes

- Losing interest in activities that were once loved

- Feeling severe fatigue or lack of energy

- Poor memory, concentration, and judgment

- Thoughts of suicide

- Preoccupation with death.

If someone you know, or even yourself, is going back and forth between signs of depression and mania, it is a major red flag for bipolar disorder. There are different types and levels of bipolar disorder. Seek out the help of a professional.

Continued research shows that targeted vagus nerve stimulation can help ease the signs and symptoms of bipolar disorder. Increasing the vagal tone through stimulation allows for an increase in calmness, and reduced anxiety and depression by calming down the nervous system. Whenever you can stimulate the vagus nerve, you can elicit the positive physiological responses that bring positive emotions. Continued research shows that harnessing the healing power of the vagus nerve has an antidepressant result and also keeps the mind from becoming overly excited.

Vagus Nerve And ADHD

ADHD is known as attention-deficit and hyperactivity disorder. It is a neurobehavioral disorder marked by a very poor attention span, coupled with hyperactivity. Many children who have ADHD have a difficult time in school and performing other activities. They may be very intelligent but being able to keep them focused is a difficult challenge. Some of the signs of ADHD include:

- Always interrupting

- Trouble waiting for their turn

- Lack of focus

- Unfinished tasks

- Daydreaming

- Trouble getting organized

- Forgetful

- Make a lot of mistakes

- Difficulty in staying quiet

Vagus nerve stimulation has been proven effective in calming the nervous system and allow improved control of emotions. This, in turn, may help to reduce the signs of ADHD and allow children to stay more focused. In many instances, medications and other medical interventions can turn children into zombies. Increasing vagal tone naturally has been shown to produce more of a neutral result. Like many other data, the research is still out on how effective vagal tone is for ADHD. At this moment, the results look promising.

As a side note, a study published in the Annals of Neuroscience published in 2016 showcases reduced heart rate variability in children with autism. This suggests a strong connection between vagal tone and the symptoms of ADHD.

Vagus Nerve And Inflammation

Inflammation is a natural immune system process that helps fight infection, illness, and injury. The immune system is responding to a threat to the body. Short-lived inflammation will not have health consequences. However, chronic inflammation will lead to many potential illnesses, like heart disease, stroke, diabetes, kidney failure, arthritis, and even some cancers. It can become quite a fatal disease process. One way to fight inflammation is through diet. Another way is by using the vagus nerve.

Since inflammation is a bodily response to stress then engaging the vagus nerve to reduce stress will also fight inflammation. The neurotransmitter acetylcholine, which is released by the vagus nerve, slows down the heart rate and reduces overall stress. This calmness that the vagus nerve brings to the body helps combat inflammation.

Chapter 6: The Keto Diet And Vagus Nerve

There is an old expression that says you are what you eat. There is some truth to this. We don't literally mean that if you eat bread, you become bread. However, what we eat plays a huge part in what we become as far as our health and well-being.

The Keto Diet

The keto diet is a high-fat low carb diet that is similar to the Atkin's diet. By reducing carb intake, your body goes into a metabolic state known as ketosis. Your body ultimately becomes very efficient at breaking down fats to gain energy, and it turns fat into ketones in the liver, which supplies energy for the brain. This diet has been shown to have a massive reduction in blood sugar levels.

There are several different types of keto diet plans. These include:

- **The standard keto diet:** This is the most common one which we described above. It boasts moderate levels of protein with the high-fat, low-carb concept.

- **Cyclical keto diet:** Allows for short periods of high carb intake. For example, you can follow the standard keto diet for five days, and then eat high-carb foods for two days straight.

- **Targeted keto diet:** Again, this diet follows the standard plan, but allows you to increase carb intake around major physical activity. For example, after a major workout session.

- **High-protein keto diet:** The standard keto diet, plus a higher percentage of proteins.

The keto diet in its various forms has been shown to have many health benefits. The standard and high-protein options have the most research behind them.

The Keto Diet And The Vagus Nerve

The keto diet and vagus nerve have been shown to have a synergistic relationship in improving health outcomes. A study published in the Epilepsies Journal in 2007 showcases a group of children who had drastic reductions in epileptic seizures when the keto diet was properly combined with vagus nerve stimulation. Also, quality of life surveys and questionnaires indicated an overall increase in mood and a decrease in mood disorders like depression and anxiety. Of course, the population of the study was quite small and much more extensive research needs to be conducted.

The vagus nerve creates a direct connection between the digestive tract and the brain. Signals run up the vagus nerve between the gut and the brain affect your perception of hunger and fullness. In addition, signals that run down the nerve from the brain to the gut affect your digestion, the release of digestive enzymes, and your gastrointestinal motility. The physical bulk of your food sends information signals up to your brain letting it know whether it is full or still has room for more. Nutrient sensing neurotransmitters can also send hunger and fullness signals to the brain via the vagus nerve.

When our vagus nerve is functioning properly, it will allow us to feel full when we are supposed, preventing us from overeating. Unfortunately, when the vagus nerve is not able to send signals properly, the information to communicate hunger and fullness becomes altered. For example, we may have eaten a full meal that would normally fill us up, but yet we still feel hungry. Our brain is telling us to eat more food to feel satiated. So, we follow the orders our brain gives to our gut and continue to eat. By the time we feel full, we may have eaten twice as much as we should have. Over time, this will lead to unhealthy weight gains and decreased energy levels.

You have noticed that in times of stress, we tend to eat more. This is because our vagus nerve is not stimulated and our sympathetic nervous system is in control. Our ability to sense how much food we are eating becomes altered. We continue to eat because our gut cannot properly communicate to the brain that we have had enough.

When we are in a state of calmness, our vagus nerve is stimulated and we have improved communication between our gut and brain. Hence, the signals for hunger and fullness and being sent up the brain more efficiently, allowing us to control our food intake. Furthermore, our digestion also improves due to an improved ability to send signals from the brain to the gut.

Many unhealthy, obesity causing diets lower the sensitivity of the vagus nerve to signals of fullness. This means when we continue to eat diets that are high in unhealthy fats, salt, sugar, and other chemicals will cause us to feel hungrier, which will result in us eating more unhealthy foods.

A healthy diet can have the reverse effect of a poor diet and increase the sensitivity in the vagus nerve. This will lead to improved communications of fullness from the gut to the brain, resulting in us eating less food. When we eat properly, we are also sending the brain information about our nutritional intake and the brain will sense that we have enough. The keto diet can provide us with the nutrition that we need for proper metabolism and energy.

The vagus nerve has a direct effect on inflammation in the body as well. Chronic inflammation can lead to severe health consequences like heart disease, kidney failure, digestive problems, respiratory issues, neurological disease, and mood disorders. Through much research, the vagus nerve has been shown to reduce inflammation by reducing the stress response, which is a major trigger for inflammation in our bodies. An increasing vagal tone will increase the efficacy of reducing inflammation. The keto diet compliments the vagus nerve once more by adding anti-inflammatory properties. Dietary fat, which is abundant in the keto diet, has been shown to reduce inflammation further through the vagus nerve.

While there is still much evidence that is needed to show the full beneficial relationship between the vagus nerve and the keto diet, much of the research suggests that there is a synergistic relationship. The keto diet essentially compliments the vagus nerve by increasing its sensitivity and viability. A healthy diet coupled with regular vagus nerve stimulation can have immense benefits on your health.

Since increased vagal tone improves the signaling between the brain and the gut, then stimulating the vagus nerve may reduce our appetite and allow us to eat less during each meal. This can be tested by utilizing some of the techniques we discussed earlier. Before eating a meal, perform deep-breathing exercises, the Valsalva maneuver, cold exposure or any number of practices to stimulate the vagus nerve. Assess whether this is causing you to become full faster and eat less with each meal.

Common Keto Foods

Certain foods are common for the Keto diet. They offer great low-carb, high-fat options. The following are some of the best foods to include in your keto diet plan.

- **Seafood:** Salmon, sardines, and mackerel are all great options as they are healthy fatty-fish. Shellfish like shrimp and crab, are also good, but just be mindful that certain types of shellfish have more carb levels than others.

- **Vegetables Low in Carbohydrates:** Most non-starchy vegetables are low-carb, so you have a wide array of options here. Starchy vegetables include potatoes, yams, or beets.

- **Cheese:** Pretty much all cheeses are low-carb and high fat, so they all fit the keto diet plan.

- **Avocados:** Avocados are one of the healthiest fats and are also full of many other nutrients.

- **Meat and Poultry:** Meat and poultry are considered a major staple in this meal plan. Fresh meat and poultry contain no carbohydrates and are filled with many other nutrients, like protein.

- **Eggs:** Eggs are very low-carb, making them very beneficial for this meal plan.

- **Coconut Oil:** Cooking with coconut oil is a positive step. It is considered a healthy fat option.

- **Plain Greek Yogurt or Cottage Cheese:** These contain a lot of protein with just a few carbohydrates.

- **Olive Oil:** This is another healthy fat used for cooking. Olives are also good.

- **Nuts and Seeds:** Good options include almonds, pecans, walnuts, pistachios, chia seeds, flaxseeds, sesame seeds, and cashews.

- **Berries:** Berries are one of the few low-carb fruits. Blackberries, blueberries, and raspberries are good options.

- **Unsweetened Coffee and Tea:** The only problem is that people load them up with sugar. However, caffeine can increase your metabolism and physical performance. Keep the coffee and tea simple by limiting creamers and sweeteners.

- **Dark Chocolate:** These are rich in antioxidants and have several anti-inflammatory properties. Dark chocolate also contains chemicals like flavanol, which has been known to reduce heart disease.

Many of these foods in the keto diet plan also help to fight inflammation, which is another way it compliments the vagus nerve.

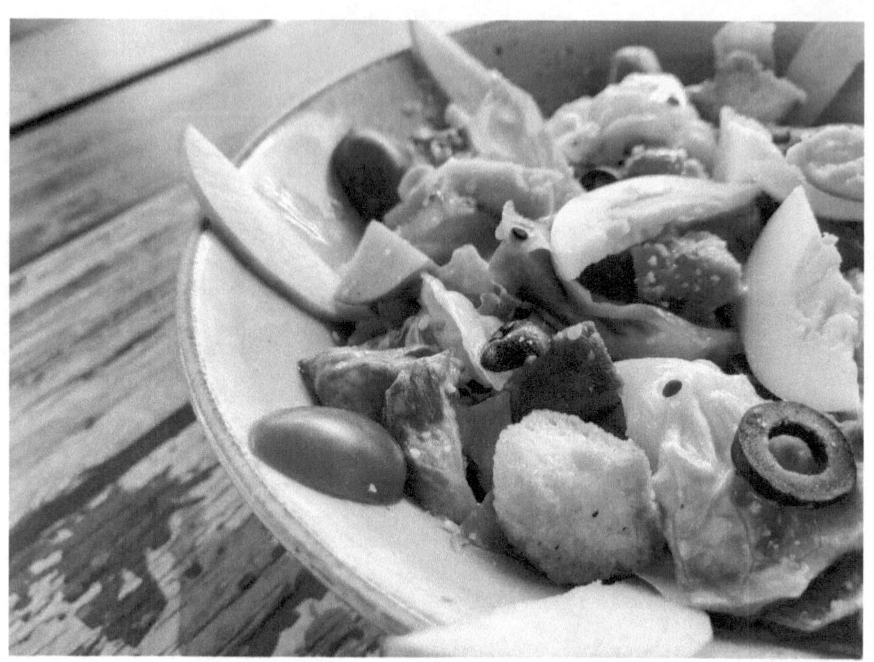

How To Begin Incorporating The Keto Diet

Since the keto diet has been shown to have many health benefits, including as a complement to the vagus nerve, we can show you ways to start incorporating it into your daily life and routine. Just like with any major change, making alterations in our diet should be done slowly so our bodies have time to adjust properly. Also, we will develop good habits in the long run.

Start by changing one of your meal plans on day one and then go up from there. Let's look at a quick sample to showcase how you can slowly incorporate the keto diet into your routine.

Monday

Breakfast: Bacon, toast with butter, and coffee with two spoons of sugar

Snack: Dark chocolate bar

Lunch: Pizza and soda

Snack: Almonds

Dinner: Large sandwich and soup

Tuesday

Breakfast: Oatmeal with green tea

Snack: Carrot sticks

Lunch: Pizza with soda

Snack: Chocolate chip cookies

Dinner: Steak

Wednesday

Breakfast: Sugary cereal and coffee

Snack: Blueberries

Lunch: Hamburger with fresh beef and cheese

Snack: Carrot sticks

Dinner: Pasta

Thursday

Breakfast: Egg white omelet with green tea

Snack: Cookies

Lunch: Greek chicken salad with a smoothie

Snack: Carrots

Dinner: Lean steak

Friday

Breakfast: Whole egg omelet with coconut oil and coffee with no sugar

Snack: Handful of almonds

Lunch: Chicken Caesar salad

Snack: Avocado

Dinner: Grilled chicken and vegetables

As we can see, over five days we were able to transition into a mostly keto diet. It does not have to be done overnight, nor should it be. Take small steps each day as the example above and you will make major progress. The sample is also only for five days. If it takes you longer, don't stress about it. As long as you are making progress every day.

We hope this book provided you all of the information you needed and ever wanted about the vagus nerve. We expect that you will use the exercises we provided for you regularly so you can also experience the amazing power of the vagus nerve. When you do, you will feel like a whole new person. You will feel better both physically and mentally. Furthermore, if you take the information you learned about the vagus nerve and couple it with a proper diet and overall healthy lifestyle, you will feel significantly different daily. You will wake up with energy, less pain, a more focused mind, and perform better overall. Finally, you will also have greater self-confidence.

Conclusion

Thank you for making it through to the end of *Vagus Nerve: From Polyvagal Theory to Self-Help Natural Exercises to Unleash Your Innate Body Power and Heal Inflammation, Anxiety, Depression, PTSD, and Autism*. Let's hope it was informative and able to provide you with all of the tools you need to achieve your goals whatever they may be. Out nervous system is one of, if not the most, critical systems in our body that controls the function of every organ, tissue, and cell in our bodies. The vagus nerve is a powerful structure and nerve that may be the most important part of our outer nervous system and behind only the brain and spinal cord in the entire network. It innervates many major areas and vital organs, so its influence in healthy and unhealthy physiological processes cannot be denied.

The vagus nerve must be taken care of regularly and stimulated to reach its full potential. When it does, the healing powers are amazing. We discussed many different methods one can use to recharge this powerful nerve. You can try just a few or all of them. The important thing is to do them regularly, whatever exercises you may choose. Many of the exercises we discussed can be done in a person's home, with just a few minutes of free time. Several research studies have suggested the idea of vagal tone as a connection to various illnesses. When vagus nerve stimulation was utilized in some form, it showed marked improvements in the signs and symptoms of various physical and mental disorders. Many of which we discussed in this book.

Once we unleash the full potential of the vagus nerve, we will not only improve our quality of life day to day but protect ourselves from many harmful diseases. This may seem like hyperbole, but the capabilities we have to take charge of our health are endless. Improve your health today by harnessing the strength of your vagus nerve.

The next step is to take the information you learned in this book and begin utilizing it in your own life. We went over many different topics related to the vagus nerve and you can start incorporating it into your daily routine as you feel comfortable. Start slow, and then progress based on your own comfort level. The more knowledge from this book that you put into practice, the more benefits you will feel.

This book is an Amazon exclusive and, if you found this book useful in any way, a review on Amazon is always appreciated!